"Suzanne Somers is the best cook I've ever known (next to my mother)! When Kari and I are invited over for one of her home-cooked meals, we never say no! Her knowledge is extraordinary. Her recipes are gastronomic magic. Not to mention, her dishes always look 'photo-ready.' A favorite? I guess that would be any of her phenomenal soups!"

—Dick Clark

"If Suzanne Somers wasn't a brilliantly talented comedic actress, she would've been a brilliantly talented gourmet chef. Having the privilege of dining at her table is a gastronomic feast I will long remember."

—Fran Drescher, actress, health advocate, hungry Jew

"More than any three-star restaurant in the world, an invitation for dinner in Suzanne's kitchen is an epicurean feast. Suzanne's cuisine is uncomplicated and of the greatest simplicity."

—Paul Bruggemans, owner of Le Vallauris Restaurant, Palm Springs

"Suzanne's cooking is outstanding. Every bite is a treasure. My favorite dish of yours is lettuce."

—Don Rickles, comedian and actor

"If you ever want to see poetry in motion, hang out in Suzanne's kitchen. Somehow, she even makes the food sexy!"

—Leeza Gibbons

"With no exaggeration, Suzanne is a master chef. From its presentation to the final bite of dessert, her cooking exceeds that of the finest restaurant in Los Angeles. My wife, Anne, and I have these favorites: lamb chops marinated in fresh herbs, garlic, and oil, pan-fried with fresh basil pesto and followed by a choice of chocolate soufflé or chocolate pot de crème. Extraordinaire."

—Arnold Kopelson, Academy Award–winning producer

"The only food I *really* look forward to is Suzanne's."

—Barry Manilow

"Suzanne can take a person who's had a lifetime of junk food and processed food (um, like me) and cook a meal so delicious, you'll just say, 'Thank you and more, please.' "

—Kathy Griffin

"You'd expect dinner with a famous health and fitness guru to taste like a porridge of tofu and library paste! But this lady can turn out a meal that will thrill your palate and be good to your body. I can't promise you'll look as good as Ms. Somers, but you'll learn that great food and great health do go together."

—Dick Van Dyke

"It's always an exciting experience to be invited to Suzanne and Alan's for dinner. Suzanne's creative imagination is reflected in the superb meals she invents. She's one sexy chef!"

—Norman Jewison, award-winning director and producer

The Sexy Forever Recipe Bible

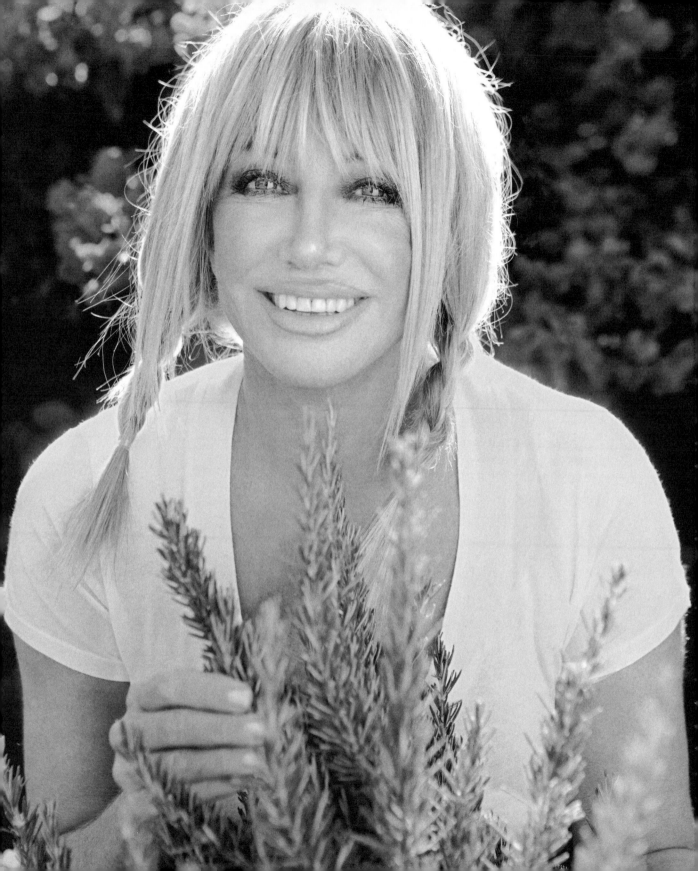

the
SEXY FOREVER
RECIPE BIBLE

suzanne somers

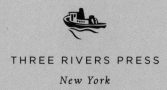

THREE RIVERS PRESS

New York

To my Somersize and Sexy Forever family:
This little girl who loved to cook grew into a woman who
somehow made a career out of it. It's a dream come true to have
all my favorite recipes in one compilation. You've been asking
for this book for years. You pulled this out of me. Each book in the
Somersize series, now Sexy Forever, has been by your request—and
none more than this one. Thank you for staying with me for all these years,
and for sharing a passion for food. I speak through my cooking.
It's how I show my love for my family and all of you.
This book is our legacy.

Library of Congress Cataloging-in-Publication Data
is available upon request.

ISBN 978-0-307-95670-5
eISBN 978-0-307-95671-2

PRINTED IN THE UNITED STATES OF AMERICA

Book design by Elizabeth Rendfleisch
Cover design by Caroline Somers and Danielle Shapero-Rudolph
Photographs by Cindy Gold

1   3   5   7   9   10   8   6   4   2

First Edition

ACKNOWLEDGMENTS

Caroline Somers, the words *thank you* don't cover enough. Caroline didn't just *help* me with this compilation, so much of it became her total responsibility. She conceptualized and produced the look of the book as well as the photographs, she took over responsibility for laying out and testing all the recipes we had created together in the other Somersize books. On a daily basis we discussed how to move forward and then she would *do* it. Lucky me. Caroline is not only my daughter-in-law, she's an invaluable part of our organization. She is protective of the brand, ensuring that all resonates with the messages of my books; in this case, how it applies to the food we eat. Caroline and I have cooked together for twenty years. She has an impeccable palate. I trust her judgment, I trust her taste, and I love her dearly.

Heather Jackson, my wonderful editor, now on our fourth book together. We have such an easy rhythm. I will find myself thinking about a revision and at the same time receive an e-mail from you with the exact same notion. We are in sync. Your help in organizing and coding this rather beastly manuscript was invaluable. I could not have met this schedule without your efforts. Thank you for your excellence and for doing it all while you were in the middle of a move, being a summer supermom, dodging a hurricane, and pitching my next big project! I love multitasking brilliant women and you are at the top of the list.

My team at Crown is like family. We have been together through it all; we've grown together through it all. I could not hope for a better, more committed publishing partner or a nicer group of professionals. We've accomplished so much throughout these years. This recipe bible wouldn't have arrived in your hands without the keen eye and cool head of Christine Tanigawa, the production editor on this as well as my last three books; or Elizabeth Rendfleisch, who epitomizes calm creativity; her interior design work is beautiful and synced so nicely with my team's vision. James Massey: thank you for your help with the cover. Thank you to Linnea Knollmueller, Luisa Francavilla, Amy Boorstein—the unseen but crucial folks behind the scenes who turn my work from words on the page into real books. And thank you to the rest of my Crown team for their hard work and evergreen support in selling, marketing, and promoting my books: Annsley Rosner, Michael Palgon, David Drake, Jill Flaxman, and Meredith McGinnis. Maya Mavjee, president and publisher, my new publisher, a great visionary with impeccable taste. I look forward to many more books in the future. Tina Constable, senior vice president and publisher of Crown Archetype, we've done so many books together and have become such good friends over the years. There is a trust and shorthand between us that is not only valuable but also a real pleasure.

Sandi Mendelson, my trusted publicist of many years. Most of my books are bestsellers. That doesn't happen unless you have a great publicity plan. Sandi is the best in the business, and she's a cool chick.

The SexyForever.com team at Everyday Health: this fabulous organization runs my online subscription program and encouraged me to write this compilation of recipes as a followup to *Sexy Forever*. While I have always wanted to do it, it was the push from Everyday Health that made it happen with Crown. I am so proud of what we have created at SexyForever.com and I know we are just beginning! Mike Keriakos, this all started as your brain child. Thank you for seeing it through. Steven Petrow, you have been my greatest cheerleader and I appreciate how you continue to champion and oversee the brand. Greg Jackson, where would we be without your commitment to advertising and marketing? Vince Errico, you conceptualize and execute each phase of development on schedule without a ruffle of your feathers. And to Sarah Hutter, Bill Maslyn, Eleanor Meyers, Margaret O'Malley, Debbie Strong, Shannon McGarity, Maggie Fabrizio, Hilary Hayward, Kelly MacDonald, and Maureen Namkoong—your daily commitment to excellence makes me proud.

Thanks to my fabulous photography team as we took off on a little scavenger hunt around Malibu for the best local ingredients. First, to the vendors who welcomed us so graciously:

Larry Thorne at Thorne Family Farms; one of my favorite times of the week is when Alan and I drive up to your organic farm to see what wonderful gifts your fertile land has sprouted. Thank you for allowing my crew to document your little slice of heaven. And thank you for the delicious food you bring to my table each week.

Nick and Stephanie Wechsler, my amazing friends with the enviable ranch that is home to llamas, cats, and Araucana chickens who lay priceless fresh eggs. Thanks for letting me feed your little babies and collect those beautiful blue, green, and pink eggs.

Malibu Seafood, our local weekend hangout and favorite spot for fresh, and I mean *fresh* seafood. I loved splashing in your crab and lobster tank. Thank you for letting us invade your store for a bit. Your energy and casual, positive vibe is as great as your fish and seafood.

Malibu Olive Company; I met Robert Jaye at the farmers' market and fell deeply, madly in love with his extra virgin olive oil. Robert, you taught me how to taste oil in beautiful blue glass (who knew color did not really matter?) and I have been a fan ever since. And thank you to Dan Romanelli for allowing us to shoot at his spectacular Tuscan villa on the beach. Wow! Simply stunning.

Diane Kron, the owner of the luscious chocolate shop KChocolatier, opened her tiny doors and allowed us to spill in and taste every delicious morsel in sight. Oh, this was a fun day of shooting! Diane, thank you for putting out such a quality product. When I tell my readers that good-quality chocolate contains antioxidants and that a small quantity will satisfy, I am speaking of chocolate like yours. Your 60% cocoa bars and wafers are essential for my chocolate baking needs—and my general addiction.

Thank you, Cindy Gold and her photography team—Paul Craig, John Guarente, and Bonnie Holland—my go-to source for the last several projects. I love the fast, easy way you shoot with natural light. No fussing for hours. This allows the real me to be reflected in these shots. To get all of these locations (including a cover shot!) in two days was simply amazing and I could not have done it with any other crew. And thank you for introducing me to Megan Fitzgerald. Oh, how I love your food styling, Megan! So real you can eat it. And we did. That shot of the chicken on the cover was the afternoon snack for the crew. And to Don Stewart for prop styling, you caught onto my clean look instantly. Thanks for your lovely restraint. Mooney, once again you are the master of hair. Thanks for coming back from Israel to get my mane back in great shape and tousling it just right. And thank you to Anna Branson for keeping my makeup fresh.

Danielle Shapero-Rudolph, thank you for another great cover design. You and Caroline make such a fabulous team, not only for this cover but also for everything in my brand. I trust your taste and appreciate the simplicity and elegance you bring to your work. Thank you for "my look" and for positively influencing the brand with your excellent eye and graphic designs. Thank you for your patience to get it just right. I also appreciate the way you interact with the talented designers at Crown to create a unified look from cover to cover.

Maria Arminio, for lending a helping hand with the recipe testing. With so many desserts, Maria tackled the chocolate, the custards, the meringues, and more to make sure our new All Natural SomerSweet was in just the right proportions. I think we got it right!

Marc Chamlin, my attorney, who keeps cranking out one book deal after the next. I love this part of my career, and thank you for assisting in keeping the work flowing.

To the women who run my life—Julie, Jordyn, and Jill. Yes, there is a theme if you want to work in my office—you must be incredibly hardworking, able to juggle many projects at once, have a superthick skin, and have a name that starts with J! You are all amazingly talented at keeping us running so smoothly, as well as being truly fine people.

Sharani and Farook: when I can't see past the manuscript in front of me, you have me pause for a bowl of soup or a rejuvenating fresh coconut with the top carved off, served with a straw and small spoon to gather the coconut milk. Thank you for the sustenance and for taking such good care of us.

And to Alan . . . it all begins and ends with you. I love you.

CONTENTS

INTRODUCTION

I love food. I have always loved food. I started cooking for my family as a young girl. I loved baking cakes. By the time I was nine, I was making beef stroganoff for the family. It was one of the few places where I had self-confidence. I was good at cooking. I received positive feedback from feeding the people I loved. That love of food almost led me to another career. After several failed TV pilots in my twenties, I had decided to give up acting. I was going to do what I knew best: cook! Life, however, doesn't always go as planned, and a little show called *Three's Company* got in the way of my cooking career. But it didn't stop my passion for food!

The Sexy Forever Recipe Bible marks my twenty-first book. You, my faithful readers, have been requesting this book for years. Many of you own some or all of my Somersize series of books with hundreds of recipes in different bindings, and you have been asking for one master book with all of them. HERE IT IS! I have taken the best of the best, revised, updated, organized, and categorized all of them to work with my amazing weight loss plan, Sexy Forever. This plan is very similar to Somersize, but with some great updates based on current science and newer discoveries related to losing weight and staying healthy.

My personal journey with weight and food began with a twiggy little body. I was one of those lucky people genetically hard-wired to be thin. Skinny. Ate whatever I wanted and didn't gain weight. Then I hit my forties, and what I didn't yet realize: the beginning of perimenopause. What were those handles on my hips? Why couldn't I hold in my stomach? And when I was trying to lose weight for the camera, why weren't the pounds flying off as they had in the past?

It wasn't until the early '90s that I discovered a weight loss program that allowed me to take off those nasty 15 pounds that had crept on in my forties, but without giving up the foods I loved. As a cook, it was a revelation to be able to lose weight and continue to eat incredible food—which has always been a huge part of the joy I find in each day. When you find a problem solver—especially something that can help others—I believe it is your duty to share it. This is how I became involved with weight loss and cookbooks.

The first of these books was published in 1996: *Eat Great, Lose Weight*. The message resonated with food lovers around the country. It was a *New York Times* bestseller. Not only were readers losing weight but, because of the recipes included in the book, they were learning to cook—and many told me they were eating the best food of their lives!

From there, "Somersize" took on a life of its own. Over the next fifteen years, I put out nine books on the subject, with more than seven hundred recipes. Plus, I developed numerous weight loss products, starting with a sweetener I could feel good about putting into my body: All Natural SomerSweet. With these recipes, millions have lost weight while cooking up a storm. And with each book, I updated the science, evolved the program, and added more delicious recipes.

My most recent book on health and weight loss, *Sexy Forever*, took the original Somersize premise, expanded it, and made it even more current by exploring the hidden obstacles to losing weight, including hormonal changes, gut health issues, and hidden food allergies. And I created an online version of the book at SexyForever.com so you can have the support you need on a daily basis. Only one thing was missing—updating the Somersize recipes to fit the revised program.

What you will notice is that none of these recipes reads like a "diet" recipe—because they aren't! Each dish starts with real food. The selection of your ingredients is the most important part of any recipe. You will see in the following pages some of my favorite spots to get real food as close to its original source as possible. I love to support local farms, farmers' markets, the neighborhood seafood market, and more. The vendors are so proud of their food, and I feel great about putting these clean, organic (whenever possible) ingredients into my recipes. And what a difference it makes in the taste! Many of the recipes are very simple because a perfectly grown tomato with olive oil and sea salt doesn't need anything else. Others require a little more time to create something special. You'll find everything you need for any given day, divided into these categories.

- Breakfasts
- Soups
- Salads
- Appetizers, Sandwiches, and Sides

- Dressings, Sauces, and Pesto
- Vegetables
- Rice, Beans, Pasta, and Grains
- Poultry
- Fish and Seafood
- Beef, Pork, and Lamb
- Desserts

Those of you following the Sexy Forever Weight Loss Plan will recognize the titles under each recipe that identify the Sexy Forever Food Groups, such as Proteins, Healthy Fats, Vegetables, Carbohydrates, and Fruit. These groups are clearly explained in *Sexy Forever*, where you learn how to eat these foods in combinations that maximize health and weight loss. In addition, the recipes identify the phases or levels of the program, from Detox (when you are just getting started) to Level 1 (weight loss) to Level 2 (maintenance). Again, for those on the program, these indicators will help you use the recipes as part of your weight loss plan.

For those of you *not* following the plan, open the book and dive in to some spectacular food! No weight loss plan is needed to enjoy the wonderful creations within. Additionally, *The Sexy Forever Recipe Bible* is not only organized with all your favorites, it also includes a coding system so you can easily identify any food to which you are allergic, any foods for which you may have an intolerance, or any foods you simply don't care to eat. Look for the following icons in the recipes.

(gf) (Gluten Free) It is now estimated that a shocking 43 percent of the population is gluten intolerant. That spectrum varies from people who are somewhat intolerant, meaning they can eat gluten only on rare occasions, all the way to those who suffer from celiac disease, the most severe form. Celiacs must avoid gluten for the rest of their lives or risk permanently damaging their intestinal lining. There is much more information on this subject in *Sexy Forever*, but the problem is so broad I felt it necessary to code the recipes here so you can enjoy incredible foods while avoiding obvious or hidden gluten. Of course, any of the recipes made with whole-grain flours may be made with a gluten-free flour of your choice. (Note: For the program, gluten-free flour is an Insulin Trigger, since it's normally made with some combination of flours from rice, corn, tapioca, etc.) I find when I cook with gluten-free flour, I need a little less (maybe 10 percent less) than regular flour. Feel free to experiment.

df (Dairy Free) For those who cannot have dairy, I have also called out hundreds of dairy-free options. Note: I do not include butter as dairy, since the milk proteins are separated out and most people can tolerate butter, even if they cannot tolerate milk. Again, adjust the recipes to your own needs.

ef (Egg Free) Since I have a severe allergy to eggs (oh, how I miss my eggs!), I have included an icon for this food. In baking, I have experimented with replacing eggs with applesauce, but I think my best results have been with milled flaxseed and water. (See details in the "Desserts" chapter.) When you combine them, it creates a gelatinous consistency; this mix works pretty well for cakes. Again, experiment and let's all share our best results!

v (Vegetarian) and **vg** (Vegan) For my numerous vegetarian friends and followers (again, there is a wide spectrum of people, some of whom eat fish and chicken and others who are much more strict about consuming animal proteins), I have identified vegetarian (no seafood, poultry, meat) and vegan options, and you will have no problem finding plenty of satisfying selections and making your own substitutions to fit your preferred lifestyle.

Throughout my life, I have tried to share my philosophy that being healthy doesn't have to feel like work. I don't diet. I don't slave away in a gym. I do make excellent food choices. Clean, tasty, real foods do not come processed in boxes or bags. They come from the earth, the sea, the field, or the farm. Choose these real foods whenever possible. When I don't or can't, I try to make up for it with supplements or by eating really well after the fact. I try not to deprive myself too much and not to indulge too much. It's a daily choice, and I know my life depends on it.

Food is thrilling. It's to be enjoyed, respected, and savored slowly. With more than four hundred recipes in this comprehensive recipe bible, you can take a journey through tastes from around the globe, from the simple and sublime to the bold and spicy. And your grateful body will thank you for choosing this high-quality, delicious food by rewarding you with a trim figure and extended longevity. Making this choice is the best recipe of all to keep you SEXY FOREVER! Enjoy.

SF (SUGAR FREE)

Why is there no icon within the recipes to indicate (sf) (Sugar Free)?

Eliminating sugar and foods that are accepted by the body as sugar is a cornerstone of my Sexy Forever Weight Loss Plan. Why then, some have asked, have I not included a code to indicate recipes that don't contain sugar? Since I don't use sugar in *any* of my recipes, there is no reason to indicate the recipes that don't include it! You can be certain that you will not find this ingredient anywhere in this book (unless you prefer to use it in place of the natural sweeteners I recommend). Just because I do not use sugar does not mean you have to give up sweet tastes. I use other sources for sweetening, and frankly, I don't even notice the difference between refined sugar and the natural sweeteners I choose.

My sweeteners of choice include organic agave nectar and All Natural SomerSweet. There has been some controversy about agave nectar recently, with some believing it has similar qualities to high-fructose corn syrup. I believe this is both an overstatement and misleading. Agave still has a much lower glycemic index than sugar and is certainly a much better choice than high-fructose corn syrup. (Agave contains fructose, which is 20 on the glycemic index, as opposed to sugar [pure glucose] which is 100.) There has also been concern about the chemicals that may be used during the manufacturing process. I always choose organic agave nectar to be certain the product is free from such chemicals.

All Natural SomerSweet is made from inulin, a naturally occurring substance found in a large number of plants, such as dandelion, wild yam, Jerusalem artichoke, onion, agave, and chicory. The natural inulin used in All Natural SomerSweet comes from chicory, which is a prebiotic fiber (2 grams per serving). Fiber is something your body needs anyway! The product also includes erythritol, another natural substance found in pears, melons, grapes, mushrooms, wine, and cheese. While categorized as a sugar alcohol, erythritol has no gassy side effects. Additionally, there is a very small amount of fructose found in our inulin blend for a small pop of sweetness, but it's such a low amount, our nutrition facts still boast 0 sugar grams per serving. Lastly, citrus peel extract adds a wonderful flavor to All Natural SomerSweet.

Best of all, it tastes, bakes, and acts like sugar, measuring spoon for spoon in coffee or tea and cup for cup in your favorite recipes. You will see it called for in many of these recipes, and feel free to try it in many more of your own. It is available in cans or portable packets at suzannesomers.com.

THE SEXY FOREVER
WEIGHT LOSS PLAN

If you've read *Sexy Forever,* you're already familiar with the precepts of the eating plan within its pages. If you haven't yet read it, please do. There are so many hidden environmental factors that could be affecting your health and waistline, and the information there is both life-saving and weight-saving. Whichever the case, I thought a brief review/refresher wouldn't hurt to have at hand while you are planning the meals you prepare from this book. And for those of you who are simply interested in fabulous recipes, dive right in and start cooking!

THE EATING PLAN

1. Eliminate Insulin Triggers and Bad Fats.
2. Commit to clean, real, organic food.
3. Choose Protein/Healthy Fats and Vegetables at most meals.
4. Eat the right Carbohydrates.

    If you are on Detox: 3 servings per day (not combined with any fats).

    If you are on Level 1: 4 servings per day (1 serving per day may be combined with a Protein/Healthy Fats and Vegetables meal).

    If you are on Level 2: Eat Carbohydrates at your discretion.

5. Eat Fruits alone, on an empty stomach.
6. Eat three meals a day, until satisfied and comfortably full. Add snacks as needed.
7. Drink eight 8-ounce glasses of water each day.
8. Wait 2 hours between meals if switching from a Carbohydrate to a Protein/Healthy Fats meal or vice versa.

THE FOOD GROUPS

PROTEINS

Eggs

Meat

Poultry

Seafood

HEALTHY FATS

Butter

Cheese

Cream

Mayonnaise

Olive oil

Sour cream

VEGETABLES

Asparagus

Broccoli

Cauliflower

Celery

Cucumber

Eggplant

Green beans

Lettuce

Mushrooms

Spinach

Tomato

Zucchini

CARBOHYDRATES
(^{1}/2 CUP = 1 SERVING)

Beans

Brown rice

Nonfat milk products

100 percent whole-grain bread, cereal, or
   pasta

Wild rice

FRUITS

Apples

Apricots

Berries

Cherries

Figs

Grapefruit

Grapes

Kiwis

Mangoes

Melons

Nectarines

Oranges

Papaya

Peaches

Pears

Pineapple

Plums

Tangerines

ELIMINATE INSULIN TRIGGERS

Alcohol

Caffeine: allow 1 cup coffee or tea a day maximum, without other food

High-insulin fruits/vegetables: bananas; beets; carrots; corn; popcorn; potatoes; pumpkins; acorn, butternut, and winter squash; sweet potatoes

Pasta made from semolina or white flour

Sugars: white sugar, brown sugar, corn syrup, honey, maple syrup, molasses

White flour

White rice

ELIMINATE BAD FATS

Corn oil

Cottonseed oil

Margarine

Partially hydrogenated vegetable oils

Peanut oil

Safflower oil

Shortening

Soybean oil

Sunflower oil

Vegetable oils

For complete food lists and more information on my revolutionary weight loss program read *Sexy Forever* or visit SexyForever.com.

breakfasts

First coffee, then....

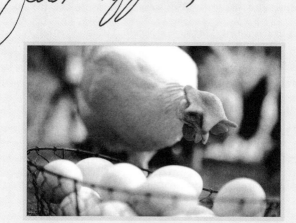

Every day begins with a choice. I wake each morning in my warm, safe bed next to Alan, my husband and partner of forty-three years. This is the gift in my life. How could I not choose to wake up feeling grateful? Any stage of life has its share of problems and angst, but I believe it's easier to choose happiness each day. Look for the good. One gift of aging is the calm that comes with it—it has given me a cool, collected approach to life. When I was younger, I often chose to be stressed and overwhelmed. With the passage of time comes wisdom and a piercing awareness of how truly blessed I am.

Of course, the fact that Alan brings me incredible coffee and a fresh-fruit smoothie in the morning certainly helps set the tone each day! After a workout, maybe yoga or some weight lifting, he makes us a full breakfast with some combination of protein, healthy fats, and/or whole-grain carbs. This is how my marriage works. He makes our morning meal, and I make dinner.

In this section, you'll find amazing recipes—many of which you can also enjoy as a lovely light lunch or dinner, like Zucchini Pancakes with Warm Tomato Coulis (page 26).

Since those of us on Sexy Forever avoid processed flour, you'll find inventive ways to make pancakes with steel-cut oats or even ricotta cheese! Plus, you have a variety of delicious egg dishes from which to choose. It starts with the selection of your egg—and all eggs are *not* created equal. Fresh, organic, cage-free eggs that slip right out of the shell are another gift, like the beautiful Araucana eggs from the chickens belonging to my friends Nick and Stephanie that were photographed for this book. Of all the organic protein I recommend, eggs are the least expensive of the bunch. If you can afford it, I highly recommend selecting the best-quality eggs you can find. (Of course, now I can only dream about these amazing egg dishes, because I have developed an allergy to these beauties!)

As for preparing the egg, this versatile gift of the food world can be transformed into so many different tasty items depending upon the numerous seasonings, vegetables, meats, or cheeses that are added, and also the type of heat used in the preparation. For instance, think about your basic scrambled eggs. If high heat is used and the eggs are stirred vigorously, you end up with brown, crumbly eggs (actually how my son, Bruce, loves them best!). With a light hand, lower heat, and more respect for the egg, you can create soft scrambled eggs with a light, dreamy texture. Alan's Fried Eggs in Onion Nests (page 12) uses olive oil and high heat to fry the eggs until they are bubbling and crispy on the edges. Divine. Our grandchildren only want their Zeda's eggs!

An omelet is the perfect way to fold vegetables, herbs, seasoning, and cheese into a sensation. Be sure to try egg cupcakes (see page 21) for an easy way to make eggs in cupcake molds—great for keeping in the freezer so you can reheat them individually on busy mornings. And a frittata just might be the ultimate brunch food. Poured into a pan and cooked, undisturbed, in a hot oven, it puffs to perfection and may be sliced and served hot; it's equally well received at room temperature. Try the Zucchini or Artichoke Frittata (pages 14 and 15)—both are definite crowd-pleasers!

However you choose to start your day, I highly recommend a good breakfast to charge your metabolism and, most important, as a moment of reflection and gratitude for the gifts in your life.

fruit smoothie

FRUIT

DETOX, LEVEL 1, LEVEL 2

Place the fruit and orange juice into a blender and process until smooth. Adjust the amount of juice to create the consistency you prefer. If you like your smoothie frozen, use frozen fruit or add a few ice cubes. Serve in wineglasses with a strawberry garnish. (*See color insert.*)   SERVES 2

1 mango, peeled and seeded, or 1 cup frozen

1 small papaya, peeled and seeded, or 1 cup frozen

$^1/_2$ cup fresh or frozen raspberries

$^3/_4$ cup orange juice

Strawberries, for garnish

Ice (optional)

fresh melon smoothie

FRUIT

DETOX, LEVEL 1, LEVEL 2

Place the melon chunks, white grape juice, and lime juice in a blender and puree until smooth and frothy. Add the ice cubes and blend until smooth. Serve immediately.   SERVES 2

2 cups seeded ripe watermelon chunks

1 cup honeydew melon chunks

$^1/_2$ cup white grape juice

Juice of 1 lime

5 or 6 ice cubes

alan's awesome bacon

PROTEIN, HEALTHY FATS

DETOX, LEVEL 1, LEVEL 2

Heat the oil in a large skillet over medium-high heat. Add the bacon and fry until golden brown, gently separating the pieces by stirring with a wooden spoon, about 7 minutes. Drain on paper towels.   SERVES 5

2 tablespoons olive oil

1 pound sliced bacon, cut into $^1/_2$-inch pieces

alan's fried eggs in onion nests

PROTEIN, HEALTHY FATS, VEGETABLES

DETOX, LEVEL 1, LEVEL 2

2 large onions

4 tablespoons olive oil

Sea salt and freshly
   ground black pepper

4 large eggs

Peel the skin off the onions and slice as thin as possible with a sharp knife, or use a mandoline to get very thin slices. In a large skillet, heat 1 tablespoon of the olive oil over medium-high heat. When the oil is hot, add the sliced onions. Let them cook until they are brown and crispy, almost burned. (Depending on your stove, this could take 10 to 15 minutes or more.) Season with salt and pepper. Scrape the onions up with a spatula and place two piles on each plate. Create the "nests" by using a fork to push out the center of each pile of onions and build up the sides.

Add the remaining 3 tablespoons olive oil to the same skillet used to cook the onions and heat over medium high. When the oil is hot, crack 2 eggs, one at a time, and drop them into the hot skillet. Let the eggs cook until the whites start to brown on the edges. Then cover the skillet with a lid and cook for 1 minute longer. When you lift the lid, the whites will be cooked all the way through and the yolks will be runny. (If you prefer the yolks cooked more, leave the lid on until the yolks are cooked to your liking.) Lift the eggs out with a spatula and place 1 egg on each onion nest. Repeat the process with the last 2 eggs.   SERVES 2

mexican omelet

PROTEIN, HEALTHY FATS, VEGETABLES
DETOX, LEVEL 1, LEVEL 2

In a medium bowl, beat the eggs and about ¼ cup water with a fork until well mixed. Add salt and pepper.

Heat a 10-inch frying pan on medium-high heat. Add half the oil and garlic. Sauté for 1 minute, then add the ground beef. Sauté the ground beef until browned. Add the spices and ¼ cup water. Turn down the heat to medium and cook until the water evaporates. Set aside.

Heat another frying pan (preferably an omelet pan) over medium to medium-high heat. To make the first omelet, add the rest of the oil and about one-fourth of the beaten eggs. You don't want the pan to be too hot or the omelet will get too brown. Let the omelet set for about 5 minutes, then, using a spatula, gently flip it over to its other side. Spoon one-fourth of the ground beef filling on top and cook for another minute. Fold the top half over the ground beef and slide onto a serving plate.

Serve immediately with a dollop of sour cream and a spoonful of salsa.

Repeat until all four omelets are completed. SERVES 4

12 large eggs

Sea salt and freshly ground black pepper

2 tablespoons olive oil (or enough to cover the bottom of the pan)

1 garlic clove, crushed

1 pound ground beef

1 teaspoon paprika

1 teaspoon ground cumin

½ teaspoon oregano

½ teaspoon chili powder

½ teaspoon cayenne pepper

Sour cream, for garnish

Salsa, for garnish

huevos rancheros

PROTEIN, HEALTHY FATS, VEGETABLES

DETOX, LEVEL 1, LEVEL 2

1 tablespoon olive oil

2 medium onions, thinly sliced

One 5-ounce can Ortega sliced chiles

1 tomato, seeded and diced

2 tablespoons (¹/4 stick) unsalted butter

4 large eggs

2 ounces sharp Cheddar cheese, grated (¹/2 cup)

Salsa, for garnish

¹/4 cup sour cream

2 scallions, white and green parts, chopped

Heat a skillet over high heat. Add the olive oil and onions. Sauté the onions until brown and crispy, about 15 minutes. Drain the chiles and add them to the onions. Add the tomato and stir until heated through. Divide onto two plates.

Add the butter to the skillet and melt it. Crack the eggs and fry them in the butter. Cover with a lid for 2 minutes to cook the whites. If you prefer the yolks cooked, cook for 1 minute longer. Repeat with the other 2 eggs.

Place 2 fried eggs on each plate over the onions. Top with the grated cheese, salsa, sour cream, and scallions.   SERVES 2

zucchini frittata

PROTEIN, HEALTHY FATS, VEGETABLES

DETOX, LEVEL 1, LEVEL 2

4 large eggs

Sea salt and freshly ground black pepper

2 tablespoons olive oil

1 medium onion, chopped

¹/2 cup julienned zucchini

Sprinkle of freshly grated Parmesan cheese

1 medium tomato, seeded and diced

10 fresh basil leaves, chopped

Preheat the oven to 350°F.

Whisk the eggs in a bowl with a splash of water. Add a dash of salt and pepper. Place a medium sauté pan (with an ovenproof handle) over medium heat. When the pan is hot, add the olive oil. Sauté the onion until crispy brown, about 15 minutes, then set aside half the onion for a garnish. Add the zucchini to the remaining onion in the hot pan and sauté for a few minutes.

Add the beaten eggs to the sauté pan.

Immediately sprinkle with the grated cheese and remove from the heat.

Place the pan in the preheated oven. (If you do not have a sauté pan with an ovenproof handle, transfer the egg mixture at this point to a small casserole dish or pie pan.) Bake for 7 to 10 minutes, until puffy and golden.

While the frittata is baking, in a separate bowl, mix the tomato, basil, and salt and pepper to taste. Top the cooked frittata with the tomato mixture and garnish with the reserved crispy onions. Slice and serve immediately or cool and serve at room temperature. SERVES 2

artichoke frittata

PROTEIN, HEALTHY FATS, VEGETABLES
DETOX, LEVEL 1, LEVEL 2

4 large eggs

Sea salt and freshly ground black pepper

2 tablespoons olive oil

2 medium onions, chopped

$^3/_4$ cup marinated artichoke hearts, drained and chopped

Sprinkle of freshly grated Parmesan cheese

Preheat the oven to 350°F.

Whisk the eggs in a bowl with a splash of water. Season with salt and pepper. Place a medium sauté pan (with an ovenproof handle) over medium heat. When the pan is hot, add the olive oil. Sauté the onions until browned and almost crispy, about 15 minutes, then set aside half the cooked onion for a garnish. Add the drained artichoke hearts and sauté for 1 minute longer.

Add the beaten eggs to the sauté pan. Immediately sprinkle with the grated cheese and remove from the heat.

Place the pan in the preheated oven. (If you do not have a sauté pan with an ovenproof handle, transfer the egg mixture at this point to a small casserole dish or pie pan.) Bake for 7 to 10 minutes, until puffy and golden. Garnish with the reserved crispy onions. Slice and serve immediately or cool and serve at room temperature. SERVES 2

grilled onion frittata

1 medium red onion, cut into 8 equal wedges

1 medium yellow onion, cut into 8 equal wedges

¼ cup olive oil

10 large eggs

¼ cup heavy cream

½ cup freshly grated Parmesan cheese

½ teaspoon sea salt

¼ teaspoon freshly ground black pepper

2 tablespoons unsalted butter

1 teaspoon finely chopped fresh rosemary

Preheat the oven to 350°F.

In a large bowl, combine the onions and olive oil and toss to coat well.

Preheat a grill or grill pan over high heat. Arrange the onion wedges on the grill and cook until browned and tender, about 5 minutes. Turn the onions over and cook until very tender, 5 to 7 minutes more. Brush with more oil as needed.

In a large bowl, beat the eggs and cream until blended. Stir in the cheese, salt, and pepper until smooth.

In a 10-inch braiser or ovenproof frying pan over medium-low heat, melt the butter. Add the rosemary and cook, stirring, for 1 minute. Pour the egg mixture into the pan and fold gently to combine rosemary and eggs. Arrange the grilled onions on top of the eggs.

Transfer the pan to the oven and bake until the frittata is golden brown and puffy, 7 to 10 minutes. Slice and serve immediately or cool and serve at room temperature. SERVES 6

spinach parmesan frittata

PROTEIN, HEALTHY FATS, VEGETABLES

DETOX, LEVEL 1, LEVEL 2

Preheat the broiler.

Break the eggs into a large bowl and beat lightly with a fork. Add the salt and pepper, nutmeg, spinach, and half the cheese and beat lightly to combine.

In a 9-inch braiser or ovenproof skillet, heat the oil over medium heat. Add the egg mixture. Reduce the heat to low and cook without stirring for about 5 minutes. There may still be some liquid on the surface at this time. Sprinkle with the remaining cheese.

Place the pan under broiler for 2 minutes or until top is puffy and golden. Remove the frittata from the broiler and let it cool in the pan for 2 minutes. Slice and serve immediately or cool and serve at room temperature. SERVES 4

6 large eggs

Sea salt and freshly ground black pepper

Freshly grated nutmeg

4 cups loosely packed fresh spinach leaves, rinsed, dried, and finely chopped

1 cup freshly grated Parmesan cheese

1 tablespoon extra virgin olive oil

feta and herb frittata

1 medium Roma (plum)
tomato

4 large eggs

1/8 teaspoon sea salt

Freshly ground black
pepper

1 tablespoon unsalted
butter

3 scallions, green parts
only, chopped

1 teaspoon chopped
fresh rosemary

1 teaspoon chopped
fresh oregano

1/3 plus 1/4 cup
crumbled feta
cheese

Preheat the broiler.

Cut the tomato lengthwise. With a teaspoon, scrape and remove seeds, then discard. Chop the tomato flesh into ½-inch pieces and set aside.

Lightly whisk the eggs in a bowl and season with the salt and pepper.

In an 8-inch frying pan with an ovenproof handle, melt the butter over medium heat. Add the tomato, scallions, rosemary, and oregano. Cook and stir for 1 minute.

Remove the pan from the heat, add egg mixture to pan, and stir to evenly distribute ingredients. Lower the heat, and sprinkle with ⅓ cup feta cheese. Cook without stirring for 5 minutes. There may still be some liquid on the surface at this time.

Place the pan under the broiler for 2 minutes or until top is puffy and golden. Remove the frittata from the broiler and let it cool in the pan for 2 minutes. Garnish with the ¼ cup feta cheese. Slice and serve immediately or cool and serve at room temperature. SERVES 2

southwestern eggs-in-a-skillet

PROTEIN, HEALTHY FATS, VEGETABLES
DETOX, LEVEL 1, LEVEL 2

Brown the sausage in a large skillet, about 5 minutes. Add the onion and cook for 5 more minutes. Add the mushrooms. Cook for an additional 5 minutes.

Drain the salsa and blend it with the sour cream. Add to the sausage mixture. Bring the mixture to a simmer, then crack the eggs on top. Cover the pan and cook on low heat for 4 minutes. Add the shredded cheese, replace the cover, and cook for 4 minutes more. Season to taste with salt and pepper. Sprinkle with cilantro and serve.   SERVES 6

1 pound chorizo
   sausage, casings
   removed and meat
   crumbled

1 large onion, chopped

6 ounces white
   mushrooms, sliced
   (about 1 cup)

1 cup fresh salsa

1 cup sour cream

6 large eggs

1 cup shredded
   Cheddar cheese

Sea salt and freshly
   ground black pepper

3 tablespoons chopped
   fresh cilantro

eggs baked in tomatoes and red peppers

PROTEIN, HEALTHY FATS, VEGETABLES

DETOX, LEVEL 1, LEVEL 2

2 tablespoons extra virgin olive oil

1 red onion, sliced

1 red bell pepper, seeded, cored, and thinly sliced

One 28-ounce can plum tomatoes, drained and chopped

Sea salt and freshly ground black pepper

4 large eggs

¼ cup crumbled feta cheese

Heat a 10-inch sauté pan on medium heat. Add the oil and onion and cook for about 5 minutes. Add the red pepper and cook for another 7 minutes. Add the tomatoes and salt and pepper to taste. Reduce heat; simmer for 30 to 40 minutes.

Creating small wells in the tomato mixture, break the eggs into the tomatoes. Cover with a lid and cook until whites have set but yolks are still runny. Sprinkle with the feta cheese and serve immediately. SERVES 2

leslie's mushroom, broccoli, and egg cupcakes

PROTEIN, HEALTHY FATS, VEGETABLES

DETOX, LEVEL 1, LEVEL 2

Preheat the oven to 350°F. Grease a 12-cup muffin tin with olive oil.

Place a large skillet over medium-high heat. Melt the butter. Add the mushrooms and sauté until they become browned and crusty on the edges, 10 to 15 minutes. Transfer the cooked mushrooms to a food processor and blend until minced. (If you don't have a food processor, you can chop the mushrooms.)

Place the broccoli florets in a steamer basket over boiling water and steam until tender, 5 to 7 minutes. Remove the broccoli from the heat and place in a mixing bowl. Add the 2 tablespoons olive oil and mash the broccoli lightly with a fork until chunky. Add the mushrooms and the grated cheese. Season with salt and pepper. Mix well with your hands.

Fill each cup half full with the mushroom-broccoli mixture.

In a bowl, beat the eggs with a splash of water until light and fluffy. Season with salt and pepper. Pour the batter into the greased cupcake tins over the vegetables until about three-quarters full.

Bake for approximately 10 minutes. Serve immediately or store each egg cup in an airtight container in the refrigerator or freezer.

MAKES ABOUT 12 EGG CUPS

2 tablespoons olive oil, plus a little for the pan

3 tablespoons unsalted butter

1 pound white mushrooms, thinly sliced

2 cups broccoli florets

6 ounces Swiss cheese, grated

Sea salt and freshly ground black pepper

10 large eggs

easy eggs florentine

PROTEIN, HEALTHY FATS, VEGETABLES

DETOX, LEVEL 1, LEVEL 2

Unsalted butter, for greasing the tin

12 thin ham slices, about 8 ounces

One 10-ounce package frozen chopped spinach, thawed and drained

Sea salt and freshly ground black pepper

12 large eggs

¾ cup finely shredded Cheddar cheese

Preheat the oven to 375°F.

Butter a 12-cup muffin tin. Press a slice of ham into each muffin cup. Divide the spinach equally among the cups, about 1 tablespoon each. Lightly season spinach with salt and pepper. Crack an egg into each cup, being careful not to break the yolk.

Bake for 10 minutes. Top each egg with 1 tablespoon grated cheese. Return to oven for an additional 5 minutes, or until the cheese has melted.

Using a heatproof spatula, carefully remove the cups from the muffin tin. Serve immediately.   SERVES 6

breakfast bruschetta

VEGETABLES, CARBOHYDRATES

DETOX, LEVEL 1, LEVEL 2

4 slices multigrain bread

2 ripe tomatoes, sliced

Sea salt and freshly ground black pepper

4 fresh basil leaves

1 sweet onion (Vidalia or Maui), thinly sliced (optional)

Toast or grill the bread until lightly browned. Top with tomato slices, salt and pepper to taste, and fresh basil leaves. Add sliced Vidalia onion rings, if desired.   SERVES 2

FOR LEVEL 1 AND LEVEL 2 Brush the grilled bread with a good-quality extra virgin olive oil.

oatmeal pancakes with blueberry sauce

PROTEIN, HEALTHY FATS, CARBOHYDRATES, FRUIT

LEVEL 1, LEVEL 2

For the pancakes: Mix all the dry ingredients. Add the milk and beaten egg white and stir until combined.

Heat a griddle to medium high. Lightly coat the griddle with grapeseed oil, then pour about ¼ cup batter per pancake onto the griddle. When the pancakes bubble on the edges, slide a spatula under them and flip.

For the blueberry sauce: Combine all the ingredients in a blender or food processor until smooth and well mixed. (Strain through a sieve if you like a smooth sauce.) Drizzle the sauce over the pancakes and serve immediately. SERVES 4

PANCAKES

$^3/_4$ cup old-fashioned rolled oats

$^3/_4$ cup whole wheat pastry flour

2 teaspoons baking powder

$^1/_2$ teaspoon baking soda

$^1/_2$ teaspoon sea salt

$1^1/_2$ cups nonfat milk

1 large egg white, beaten

Grapeseed or coconut oil, for greasing the pan

BLUEBERRY SAUCE

2 cups fresh blueberries or 1 package frozen

1 teaspoon fresh lemon juice

$^1/_2$ cup nonfat yogurt (optional, for a creamier sauce)

irish oatmeal pancakes with raspberry sauce

PROTEIN, HEALTHY FATS, CARBOHYDRATES, FRUIT

LEVEL 1, LEVEL 2

1¹/₂ cups cooked McCann's Irish Oatmeal (steel-cut oats) or quick-cooking oats

1 cup nonfat yogurt

¹/₂ cup nonfat milk

1 large egg white, lightly beaten

1 teaspoon baking soda

¹/₂ teaspoon sea salt

1 teaspoon vanilla extract

¹/₄ cup All Natural SomerSweet

Grapeseed or coconut oil, for greasing the pan

Raspberry Sauce (recipe follows)

Place the oats, yogurt, milk, egg white, baking soda, salt, vanilla, and All Natural SomerSweet in a mixing bowl. Stir until well blended. Allow to stand for 5 minutes.

Heat a griddle to medium high. Lightly coat the griddle with oil, then pour a scant ¼ cup batter per pancake onto the griddle. Cook for 2 to 3 minutes, or until golden brown, then flip with a spatula and cook for a minute more. Serve with raspberry sauce. SERVES 4

raspberry sauce

CARBOHYDRATES, FRUIT

LEVEL 1, LEVEL 2

6 ounces fresh raspberries (about 1 cup)

¹/₄ cup nonfat yogurt

¹/₂ cup All Natural SomerSweet

Bring the raspberries and 1 cup water to a boil in a small saucepan over medium-high heat. Turn heat to low and simmer for 15 minutes. Place the mixture in a sieve set over a bowl. Allow the mixture to drain, pressing lightly on the pulp to extract all the juices. Add the yogurt and All Natural SomerSweet. Stir until the All Natural SomerSweet has dissolved. Serve over the pancakes. MAKES 1¹/₂ CUPS

cream cheese pancakes

PROTEIN, HEALTHY FATS

LEVEL 1, LEVEL 2

For the pancakes: In a medium bowl, mix the cream cheese, egg yolks, All Natural SomerSweet, and cinnamon until well blended.

In another bowl, beat the egg whites with an electric mixer until stiff peaks form. Fold the egg whites into the cream cheese mixture.

Heat a griddle to medium and add a little butter. Spoon about ⅓ cup of the batter onto the griddle. Cook until golden brown, 2 to 3 minutes. Flip and cook other side to a golden brown, adding butter to the griddle as needed.

For the SomerSweet syrup: Mix the All Natural SomerSweet with the melted butter until dissolved. Stir in the cinnamon and pour over pancakes. SERVES 4 TO 6

PANCAKES

One 8-ounce package cream cheese

4 large eggs, separated

2½ teaspoons All Natural SomerSweet

½ teaspoon ground cinnamon

Unsalted butter, for the griddle

SYRUP

3 tablespoons All Natural SomerSweet

4 tablespoons (½ stick) unsalted butter, melted

½ teaspoon ground cinnamon

ricotta pancake

PROTEIN, HEALTHY FATS, CARBOHYDRATES

DETOX, LEVEL 1, LEVEL 2

Place the ricotta in a medium bowl and add the eggs, one at a time, stirring well after each addition. Add the fennel, salt, and pepper.

Heat the olive oil briefly in a large skillet over medium heat. Pour in the egg-ricotta mixture to make one large pancake. Gently move the mixture around with a wooden spoon until the egg sets, 5 to 6 minutes. The surface will still be a little runny. Invert the pancake onto a plate, cooked side up. Then slide the pancake back into the skillet to cook the other side for 1 to 2 minutes more. Slice into four wedges and serve immediately. SERVES 4

1½ cups whole milk ricotta cheese

4 large eggs

1 teaspoon fennel seeds

Sea salt and freshly ground black pepper

1 tablespoon olive oil

zucchini pancakes with warm tomato coulis

PROTEIN, HEALTHY FATS, VEGETABLES

DETOX, LEVEL 1, LEVEL 2

TOMATO COULIS

3 tablespoons olive oil

1 medium onion, diced

2 garlic cloves, minced

3 large ripe tomatoes, peeled, seeded, and diced, or 6 canned Italian plum tomatoes, seeded

5 dried bay leaves

1 teaspoon chopped fresh thyme

Sea salt and freshly ground black pepper

ZUCCHINI PANCAKES

1 large zucchini, shredded

3 large eggs

3 tablespoons chopped flat-leaf parsley

$3/4$ teaspoon sea salt

$1/2$ teaspoon ground white pepper

2 tablespoons ($1/4$ stick) unsalted butter

Freshly grated Parmesan cheese, for garnish

For the coulis: Heat the oil in a medium skillet over moderate heat. Add the onion and sauté until golden brown, about 15 minutes. Add the garlic and sauté for 1 minute more. Add the tomatoes, bay leaves, thyme, salt, and pepper. Reduce to a simmer and cook uncovered for 15 minutes. Remove the bay leaves. Keep warm.

For the pancakes: Preheat the broiler. In a bowl, mix the zucchini with the eggs, parsley, salt, and pepper.

Melt 1 tablespoon of the butter in a small ovenproof skillet over medium-high heat. (If you have two skillets, use both at the same time, one for each pancake. If you don't, keep the first pancake in a warm oven while you make the second.) Add half of the zucchini mixture and reduce the heat to low. Gently cook for 3 to 5 minutes, shaking the pan occasionally. The pancake should be loose in the center but set around the edges. Transfer the skillet to the broiler. Cook until firm in the center, about 4 minutes. (If you don't have a skillet with an ovenproof handle, you can flip the pancake by inverting it onto a plate, browned side up. Then slide it back into the skillet to cook the other side.) Repeat for second pancake.

Slice each pancake into three wedges and center on serving plates. Garnish with the tomato coulis and sprinkle with Parmesan cheese. Serve immediately. SERVES 6

zucchini muffins

VEGETABLES, CARBOHYDRATES

DETOX, LEVEL 1, LEVEL 2

Preheat the oven to 400°F. Lightly oil two 12-cup muffin tins.

Heat the milk in a medium saucepan until just boiling. Add the All Natural SomerSweet, vanilla and orange extracts, cinnamon, and nutmeg. Remove from heat and set aside.

In a large mixing bowl, combine the oats, All-Bran, zucchini, and yogurt. Add the hot milk and mix to form a batter. Stir in the flour, and add the baking powder, baking soda, lemon zest, lemon juice, and orange zest. Stir well.

Scoop the batter into the muffin tins. Bake at 400°F for 8 minutes, then reduce the heat to 350°F and bake for an additional 20 to 25 minutes, or until golden brown.

When the muffins have cooled, store those that will not be eaten within a day or two individually in an airtight container, and freeze.   MAKES 24 MUFFINS

NOTE All-Bran may contain sugar but only trace amounts, which will not create an imbalance.

Grapeseed or coconut oil, for greasing the pan

2$^1\!/_2$ cups nonfat milk

$^3\!/_4$ cup All Natural SomerSweet

2 tablespoons vanilla extract

1 tablespoon orange extract

$^1\!/_4$ teaspoon ground cinnamon

$^1\!/_4$ teaspoon grated nutmeg

2 cups quick-cooking oats

2 cups All-Bran cereal (see Note)

2 medium zucchini, shredded (about 2 cups)

32 ounces nonfat plain yogurt

4 cups whole wheat flour

2$^1\!/_2$ teaspoons baking powder

2$^1\!/_2$ teaspoons baking soda

1 teaspoon grated lemon zest

2 tablespoons plus 2 teaspoons lemon juice

3 tablespoons grated orange zest

soups
a Cup of Comfort

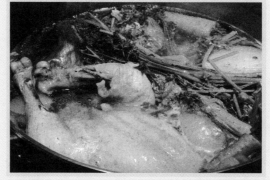

Stranded on a deserted island and you can only pick one food to eat for the rest of your life . . . Ever played this game? My answer is "chicken soup." It's the perfect food. Comforting, warm, nourishing, and delicious.

Any good cook knows your soup or sauce is only as good as your broth. I make broth about once a week, and keep it in the freezer to use as needed. A meaty carcass and some vegetable trimmings are all you need. All week I gather them in a baggie in the freezer: chicken bones, ends of carrots and celery, parsley stems, kale stems. Nothing is wasted. Then I toss them into a pot with water and cook them down to a golden broth.

You'll find several versions of chicken soups, stock, and broth. (I am often asked what the difference is between stock and broth. Quite simply, stock is unseasoned and broth has added salt.) Using a whole, raw chicken will give you a cleaner, clearer broth. A roasted chicken carcass (don't forget to include the scraped bits from the bottom of the pan) will provide a heartier, richer broth.

The peasant housewife method of cooking means not wasting any ingredients, and that's a virtue we should all live by. I taught my son, Bruce, to make a chicken last a week when I sent him off to college: Roast a chicken on Sunday night. Enjoy your dinner, then pull off any extra meat. Use the carcass to make stock for soup. The leftover chicken will provide dinner on Monday, with extra for sandwiches or salads. Then use your stock to make soup to enjoy for the next couple of days. Now one dinner lasts all week long.

Once you have broth (chicken, vegetable, beef, etc.), making soup is a snap. Try the Chicken Tomato Cilantro Soup (page 38) for an easy South American taste. Toss in soy sauce and bok choy for Asian Turkey Meatball Soup (page 38). Make delicious "egg" noodles with no flour for a traditional Jewish grandmother's soup (page 30). I love Tom Yum Kai (page 39) with the Thai flavor explosions of lemongrass, lime leaf, and chiles. Or go Italian with Stracciatella Soup (page 36) with egg ribbons and spinach.

Have your ladle ready. Soup warms the soul . . . and everyone always wants more.

grandma's traditional chicken soup

STOCK

One 4-pound chicken, or meaty chicken carcass

1 medium onion, halved

3 celery stalks, roughly chopped

3 carrots, roughly chopped (omit for Detox)

Stems from 1 bunch flat-leaf parsley

Handful of whole black peppercorns (approximately 25)

SOUP

5 celery stalks, chopped

5 carrots, peeled and chopped (omit for Detox)

3 leeks, cleaned well and chopped

1 bunch flat-leaf parsley, chopped

Sea salt and freshly ground black pepper

For the stock: Place the chicken or chicken carcass into a large stockpot. Add the remaining stock ingredients. Fill with water to cover and cook over high heat until it comes to a boil. Turn the heat to low and simmer for about 4 hours. Strain the stock, discarding the vegetables but reserving the carcass. Place the stock into a container and refrigerate. When the stock is chilled, skim off the fat that has risen to the top.

Pick the meat off the chicken, being careful to discard any bones, skin, fat, and tendons. (This is a tedious process but well worth the effort.) Reserve the meat.

For the soup: Reheat the defatted chicken stock in a large pot. Add the celery, carrots, leeks, parsley, and any chicken meat. Cook until vegetables are tender, about 20 minutes over medium heat. Season to taste with salt and pepper. SERVES 6

FOR LEVEL 2 Add 1 cup cooked wild rice to the soup just before serving.

roasted chicken stock

PROTEIN, VEGETABLES

DETOX, LEVEL 1, LEVEL 2

One 6-pound roasting chicken, with giblets

4 celery stalks, with tops

1 large onion, cut in half

4 sprigs fresh thyme

1 tablespoon fresh rosemary leaves

Sea salt and freshly ground black pepper

1 cup dry white wine (use water for Detox)

1 bunch flat-leaf parsley

Preheat the oven to 500°F.

Remove the giblets and neck from the cavity of the chicken and put them in a roasting pan. Rinse the bird and stuff the large cavity with celery stalks and half the onion. Place the other onion half under the tail flap. Stuff the thyme and rosemary under the skin of the breast.

Sprinkle the bird with salt and pepper and roast for 10 minutes. Lower the oven temperature to 325°F and continue to roast for 1 hour 50 minutes (20 minutes per pound). Remove the chicken and set it aside.

Carefully pour the contents of the roasting pan (the neck, giblets, and pan drippings) into an 8-quart stockpot. Be sure to get every last bit off the bottom of the roasting pan. Add all the remaining ingredients to the stockpot along with 12 cups of water and let come to a boil.

Remove the skin from the chicken and discard. Remove large pieces of meat and put away for later. Split the bones with a mallet and add to the stock. Bring the stock back to a boil, being careful to skim off any foam that comes to the top. Simmer the stock for about 4 hours.

Strain the stock through a fine sieve. Discard the bones and vegetables. Store the stock in containers in the refrigerator or freezer. Remove the fat after it solidifies.

MAKES ABOUT 10 CUPS

FOR LEVEL 2 Add 2 or 3 carrots for extra flavor.

incredible chicken wing broth

PROTEIN, VEGETABLES

DETOX, LEVEL 1, LEVEL 2

5 pounds chicken wings

1 head garlic, unpeeled

2 leeks, washed and cut into thirds

5 shallots, peeled

8 celery stalks (including leaves), cut into thirds

Sea salt to taste

20 black peppercorns

3 sprigs fresh thyme

1 bunch flat-leaf parsley

Place all the ingredients in a stockpot and add water to cover. Bring to a boil, then turn down to lowest heat. Cover and simmer on the lowest possible setting for about 3 hours.

Strain the broth and discard all other ingredients. Put the broth in the refrigerator and let fat harden on top, about 4 hours. Skim the fat off the top when cooled, and discard.   MAKES 2 QUARTS

quick rich broth

PROTEIN, VEGETABLES

DETOX, LEVEL 1, LEVEL 2

One 5- to 6-pound chicken

1 veal bone

1 beef bone

1 piece pancetta

1 bunch celery, cut into pieces

1 red onion

2 tomatoes

1 head garlic, unpeeled

6 dried bay leaves

6 sprigs fresh thyme

1 teaspoon black peppercorns

Sea salt

Remove any fatty parts of the chicken. Rinse the bird and place in a large stockpot with all the other ingredients except the salt, and add 8 cups water. Bring to a gentle boil over medium-high heat. Turn down the heat and skim any foam from the top. Simmer for about 1 hour. Strain the broth through a fine sieve. Remove the chicken and set aside for another meal. Discard the meat and vegetables.

Season with salt. Store the broth in containers in the refrigerator or freezer. When the broth is thoroughly chilled, fat will rise to the top and harden. Remove all the fat and discard.   MAKES ABOUT 8 CUPS

FOR LEVEL 2 Add 2 carrots for extra flavor.

vegetable stock

VEGETABLES

DETOX, LEVEL 1, LEVEL 2

In a large stockpot, combine all the ingredients and 8 cups of water and bring to a boil. Reduce the heat and simmer for 3 hours. Strain and discard the vegetables and peppercorns.   MAKES ABOUT 6 CUPS

FOR LEVEL 2 Add 5 carrots for extra flavor.

2 heads garlic, unpeeled

4 medium onions, halved

5 leeks, washed and roughly chopped

1 bunch flat-leaf parsley

1 bunch thyme

5 dried bay leaves

5 celery stalks

25 black peppercorns

roasted vegetable stock

VEGETABLES

DETOX, LEVEL 1, LEVEL 2

Preheat the oven to 350°F.

Place the red pepper, celery, onion, turnips, parsnip, and rutabaga in a baking dish. Sprinkle with the salt. Place the dish in the oven and roast the vegetables for 30 minutes.

Place the roasted vegetables, 8 cups of water, and all the remaining ingredients into a stockpot. Make sure you scrape all the bits from the baking dish. Simmer for 1½ hours.

Strain the stock through a fine sieve, making sure to squeeze the juice out of the vegetables. Discard the vegetables.

MAKES ABOUT 6 CUPS

FOR LEVEL 2 Add 2 carrots for extra flavor.

1 red bell pepper

4 celery stalks, with tops

1 medium sweet onion (Vidalia or Maui)

2 small turnips

1 small rutabaga

1 tablespoon sea salt

3 garlic cloves

1 leek

1 cup dry white wine (omit for Detox)

1 bunch flat-leaf parsley

8 sprigs fresh thyme

10 black peppercorns

1 teaspoon paprika

beef stock

2 beef shanks

4 large short ribs

1 tablespoon sea salt

1 cup dry red wine (use water for Detox)

4 celery stalks, with tops

1 medium onion

4 garlic cloves

10 black peppercorns

2 sprigs fresh thyme

1 sprig fresh rosemary

Preheat the oven to 350°F.

Season the beef shanks and short ribs with the salt and place in a roasting pan. Roast for 30 minutes. Remove the shanks and ribs and place in a large stockpot. Place the roasting pan on the stove over medium-high heat. When the pan is hot, add the wine and continue stirring, scraping the bits off the bottom of the pan to release the flavor. Pour the contents of the roasting pan into the stockpot.

Add all the other ingredients and 6 cups of water, and cook over medium-low heat. The stock should cook for 3 to 5 hours.

Strain the stock through a fine sieve. Discard the meat and vegetables. Store the stock in containers in the refrigerator or freezer. When the stock is thoroughly chilled, fat will rise to the top and harden. Remove all the fat with a spatula.   MAKES ABOUT 10 CUPS

FOR LEVEL 2 Add 2 or 3 carrots for extra flavor.

fish broth

2 fresh fish heads and tails

1 cup dry white wine (omit for Detox)

1 leek, washed and cut in half lengthwise

2 celery stalks

1 tablespoon paprika

1 tablespoon sea salt

Combine all the ingredients, except the salt, and 8 cups of cold water in a stockpot and place over medium-low heat. Bring to a simmer, not a boil. Let simmer for 2 to 3 hours. Drain the broth through a fine sieve, then discard the fish and vegetables. Add the salt. Store the broth in containers in the refrigerator or freezer.   MAKES ABOUT 6 CUPS

egg crêpe noodles in chicken broth

PROTEIN, HEALTHY FATS, VEGETABLES

DETOX, LEVEL 1, LEVEL 2

To make the egg crêpes into noodles, roll up each crêpe, then slice into noodles approximately ½ inch wide. (If they are too narrow, they tend to disintegrate in the hot soup.)

Fill soup bowls with the hot broth and add a handful of noodles just before you serve. Season to taste with salt and pepper. Garnish with the parsley. SERVES 4

4 to 6 Egg Crêpes (recipe follows)

4 cups chicken stock or broth, preferably homemade (pages 30–32), heated

Sea salt and freshly ground black pepper

½ cup chopped flat-leaf parsley

egg crêpes

PROTEIN, HEALTHY FATS

DETOX, LEVEL 1, LEVEL 2

6 large eggs

Sea salt and freshly ground black pepper

Melted unsalted butter

In a mixing bowl, lightly beat the eggs. Season with salt and pepper. Heat a crêpe or omelet pan over medium to medium-high heat and lightly coat the bottom and sides with butter.

Using a ladle, put just enough egg in the pan to make a thin coating. When it sets, lift up with a spatula, being careful not to tear the crêpe, and flip. Cook 1 minute more, then slide the crêpe out of the pan and onto a dish. Continue making egg crêpes in this way until you have used all the batter. Stack the crêpes as you would pancakes. MAKES ABOUT 8 CRÊPES

stracciatella soup

PROTEIN, HEALTHY FATS, VEGETABLES

DETOX, LEVEL 1, LEVEL 2

4 cups chicken stock or broth, preferably homemade (pages 30–32)

6 ounces fresh spinach or frozen spinach, thawed and drained

2 large eggs, lightly beaten

Sea salt and freshly ground black pepper

1/4 cup freshly grated Parmesan cheese

Bring the chicken stock to a boil in a large pot. Add the spinach and simmer for about 4 minutes. Quickly stir in the beaten eggs, and continue to stir vigorously until eggs have coagulated and turned white.

Ladle into soup bowls. Season to taste with salt and pepper. Spoon Parmesan cheese on top and serve immediately. SERVES 4

chicken meatball–asparagus soup

PROTEIN, HEALTHY FATS, VEGETABLES

DETOX, LEVEL 1, LEVEL 2

9 to 10 tablespoons olive oil

1 medium onion, chopped

1 large bunch asparagus, thinly sliced, washed and tough lower stems removed

5 leeks, white part only, washed and thinly sliced

6 cups chicken stock or broth, preferably homemade (pages 30–32)

1 pound ground chicken

Sea salt and freshly ground black pepper

Heat a stockpot over medium-high heat. Add 3 tablespoons olive oil. Add the onion and sauté until light brown, 7 to 10 minutes. Add the asparagus and leeks; sauté another 5 minutes. Add the chicken stock and bring to a boil, then reduce the heat and simmer for about 15 minutes.

Meanwhile, mix the ground chicken with salt and pepper. Make small meatballs, about 1 inch in diameter. In a 10-inch skillet, heat the remaining 6 to 7 tablespoons olive oil and fry the meatballs until browned on all sides. Add the meatballs to the soup and serve. Adjust the seasoning as needed. SERVES 4

chicken sausage and spinach soup

PROTEIN, HEALTHY FATS, VEGETABLES
DETOX, LEVEL 1, LEVEL 2

Remove fresh sausage meat from casing and form into 1-inch balls. (If using cooked sausage, cut into ¼- inch slices.)

Heat the butter and oil in a large, heavy pot over medium-high heat. Add the sausage and fry until browned, about 7 minutes. Add the chicken stock. Bring to a boil, reduce the heat, and simmer until the sausage is cooked through, about 12 minutes.

Add the spinach and simmer for 1 minute. Season to taste with salt and pepper. Serve with Parmesan cheese. SERVES 6

1 pound fresh or cooked sweet Italian chicken or turkey sausage

1½ tablespoons unsalted butter

1½ tablespoons olive oil

6 cups chicken stock or broth, preferably homemade (pages 30–32)

One 10-ounce package frozen whole-leaf spinach, thawed and drained

Sea salt and freshly ground black pepper

Freshly grated Parmesan cheese, for garnish

chicken tomato cilantro soup

PROTEIN, HEALTHY FATS, VEGETABLES

DETOX, LEVEL 1, LEVEL 2

8 cups chicken stock or broth, preferably homemade (pages 30–32)

One 28-ounce can Italian plum tomatoes, with juice

1 teaspoon dried oregano

2 cups leftover chicken pieces

Sea salt and freshly ground black pepper

6 tablespoons chopped fresh cilantro

Heat the chicken stock in a large stockpot.

Roughly chop the tomatoes and add them to the stock along with their juice. Add the oregano, leftover chicken, and salt and pepper to taste. Simmer over medium heat for 30 minutes, then serve the soup hot, with a sprinkle of cilantro.   SERVES 6

asian turkey meatball soup

PROTEIN, HEALTHY FATS, VEGETABLES

DETOX, LEVEL 1, LEVEL 2

6 cups chicken stock or broth, preferably homemade (pages 30–32)

1 pound ground turkey, rolled into 1-inch balls

2 celery stalks, finely chopped

5 slices fresh ginger, peeled

2 tablespoons soy sauce, plus more to taste

1/2 teaspoon hot chili oil, plus more to taste

2 heads baby bok choy

Bring the stock to a boil and add the turkey balls a few at a time. Stir to ensure they do not stick together. Then add the celery, ginger, soy sauce, and chili oil. Reduce the heat and simmer for 30 minutes. Add the bok choy and simmer for an additional 5 minutes. Adjust the flavor with additional soy sauce and chili oil. Serve immediately.   SERVES 4

tom yum kai—spicy thai chicken soup

PROTEIN, HEALTHY FATS, VEGETABLES

DETOX, LEVEL 1, LEVEL 2

Heat the chicken stock in a stockpot. Add the lemongrass, lime leaves, chiles, fish sauce, ginger, and galangal. Lower the heat and simmer for 30 minutes or more. Once the stock has been infused with the seasonings, strain it, since the lemongrass, lime leaves, ginger, and galangal are for flavoring the stock, not for eating.

Add the chicken, tomatoes, cilantro, mushrooms, and lime juice. Simmer an additional 30 minutes, then serve.   SERVES 6

NOTE When working with chiles, wear kitchen gloves while washing, cutting, and seeding them. When you are finished, thoroughly wash the gloves with hot water and soap. Avoid any direct contact with the eyes while preparing chiles.

8 cups chicken stock or broth, preferably homemade (pages 30–32)

3 stalks lemongrass, cut into large pieces

1/4 cup kaffir lime leaves

2 to 5 serrano chiles (see Note)

1/4 cup Thai fish sauce (nam pla)

12 slices peeled fresh ginger

6 slices peeled galangal

Two 6-ounce skinless and boneless chicken breasts, cut into bite-size pieces

12 cherry tomatoes, halved

1/2 cup coarsely chopped cilantro

One 16-ounce can straw mushrooms, drained

Juice from 2 limes

turkey and shiitake mushroom soup

2 tablespoons olive oil

2 onions, chopped

1 pound fresh shiitake or white button mushrooms, thinly sliced

Sea salt and freshly ground black pepper

1 tablespoon chopped fresh tarragon

2 pounds ground dark turkey

1/4 cup dry white wine (use water for Detox)

1 tablespoon unsalted butter

1/2 cup sliced celery

6 cups chicken stock or broth, preferably homemade (pages 30–32)

2 medium zucchini, cut into bite-size pieces

1/4 cup freshly grated Parmesan cheese, for garnish (optional)

Place a large pot over high heat. Add the olive oil and onions, and stir constantly until the onions start to brown. Turn down the heat to medium and continue stirring until the onions are a deep golden brown and begin to caramelize, about 15 minutes. Add the mushrooms, then season with salt and pepper and the tarragon. Stir constantly until the mushrooms get brown and crusty, 15 to 20 minutes.

Add the ground turkey a little at a time, using your fingers to break it up. Add additional salt and pepper. Brown the meat for about 5 minutes, stirring constantly. Pour in the wine and cook until the steam subsides and the alcohol is burned off, another 5 minutes. Scrape the browned bits off the bottom of the pan to release the flavors. Add the butter and celery, stirring to combine. Add the chicken stock. Bring to a boil, then lower the heat and let the soup simmer for about 15 minutes. Add the zucchini and simmer 5 minutes more.

Serve in soup bowls, with freshly grated Parmesan cheese, if desired. SERVES 8

lobster bisque cappuccino

PROTEIN, HEALTHY FATS, VEGETABLES, CARBOHYDRATES,
INSULIN TRIGGERS

LEVEL 2

One 1$\frac{1}{2}$- to 2-pound
lobster, cooked (with
the shell)

4 tablespoons ($\frac{1}{2}$ stick)
unsalted butter

1 onion, sliced

1 celery stalk, sliced

1 red bell pepper,
seeded, cored, and
sliced

2 tablespoons tomato
paste

2 cups dry white wine

4 cups chicken stock
or broth, preferably
homemade
(pages 30–32)

2 cups heavy cream

Sea salt and freshly
ground black pepper

1 cup nonfat milk or
heavy cream

Remove the lobster meat from the tails and claws and set aside. Reserve the lobster shells.

Place a stockpot over medium heat. Add 1 tablespoon of the butter, the onion, celery, and red pepper. Cook for about 10 minutes to let the vegetables slowly sweat. Add the lobster shells to the pot, mashing with a wooden spoon to break up the shells and release the flavor. Add the tomato paste, stirring with the shells until it begins to caramelize.

Add the wine to deglaze the pan. Bring to a boil, then lower the heat to a simmer and reduce by half. Add the chicken stock and cook over medium heat until it boils. Then lower the heat to a simmer for 10 minutes. Add the cream and still at a simmer reduce the entire soup again by half.

Strain the soup through a medium sieve, pressing the shells and vegetables to extract all the flavor. Pour the strained liquid into a large pot and bring back to a simmer. Adjust the seasoning with salt and pepper. Using a whisk, incorporate the remaining 3 tablespoons of butter.

Using a milk frother, foam the milk until light and fluffy. (If you do not have a milk frother, whip a small amount of heavy cream to soft peaks instead.)

To serve as a tray-passed appetizer, fill demitasse cups two-thirds full, top with a piece of lobster meat and dollop of foamed milk, and serve immediately. To serve as a first course at a sit-down dinner, cut up the lobster meat into small chunks and place a few chunks of meat in each serving cup. Add the bisque until the cup is two-thirds full and top with a dollop of foamed milk. Serve immediately. SERVES 8

crab bisque with sweet corn and crab relish

PROTEIN, HEALTHY FATS, VEGETABLES, INSULIN TRIGGERS

LEVEL 2

1 tablespoon butter

1 onion, sliced

1 celery stalk, sliced

1 red bell pepper, seeded and sliced

1 whole Dungeness crab, steamed whole and peeled, $\frac{1}{2}$ cup crabmeat reserved for the relish

2 tablespoons tomato paste

2 cups dry white wine

4 cups chicken stock or broth, preferably homemade (pages 30–32)

2 cups heavy cream

2 ears fresh corn, kernels removed and reserved for the relish

Sweet Corn and Crab Relish (recipe follows)

Place a large stockpot over medium heat. Add the butter, onion, celery, and red pepper and cook for about 10 minutes to let the vegetables slowly sweat. Add the crab shells to the pot, mashing with a wooden spoon to break up the shells and release the flavor. Add the tomato paste, stirring with the shells until it begins to caramelize.

Add the wine to deglaze the pan. Bring to a boil, then lower the heat to a simmer and reduce by half. Add the chicken stock and cook over medium heat until it boils. Then lower the heat to a simmer for 10 minutes. Add the cream and still at a simmer reduce the entire soup again by half.

Strain through a medium sieve, pressing the shells and vegetables to extract all the flavor. Pour the strained bisque into a clean pot and add the corn cobs and any crabmeat not used for the relish. Cook on low for 5 to 8 minutes, until the bisque is thickened. Remove the corn cobs. Ladle into soup bowls and garnish with a generous spoonful of the sweet corn and crab relish. (*See color insert.*)   SERVES 4

sweet corn and crab relish

PROTEIN, VEGETABLES, INSULIN TRIGGERS

LEVEL 2

1^1/$_2$ cups corn kernels

^{1}/$_2$ cup lump crabmeat

1 jalapeño chile, seeded and finely diced (see Note, page 39)

1 tablespoon chopped flat-leaf parsley

Juice from ^{1}/$_2$ lemon

1 shallot or ^{1}/$_4$ red onion, finely diced

Sea salt and freshly ground black pepper

If using ears, slice the kernels off the cobs. (Reserve the cobs to flavor the crab bisque.) Toss all the ingredients in a bowl. Serve immediately or store in an airtight container in the refrigerator. MAKES 2 CUPS

fennel soup with ricotta whole wheat bruschetta

PROTEIN, HEALTHY FATS, VEGETABLES, CARBOHYDRATES

LEVEL 1, LEVEL 2

4 medium fennel bulbs

4 cups chicken stock or broth, preferably homemade (pages 30–32)

Sea salt and freshly ground black pepper

6 slices crusty whole wheat bread

1 garlic clove, split in half

12 tablespoons skim-milk ricotta cheese

Extra virgin olive oil, for drizzling

Freshly grated Parmesan cheese, for garnish

Slice a few of the feathery leaves from the tops of the fennel and set aside. Cut the stems off the fennel, leaving just the bulbs. Cut off any brown part on the bottom of the bulbs. Remove and discard any tough or bruised outer layers and slice the bulbs into ½-inch pieces.

Bring the stock to a boil and add the fennel. Cook until tender, about 20 minutes. Add a few chopped fennel leaves and season with salt and pepper.

Grill or toast the bread slices. While still hot, rub the toast with the garlic clove. Spread 2 tablespoons ricotta over each piece of toast and place a piece in each soup bowl.

Spoon the cooked fennel over the bread, then ladle in some of the stock. Drizzle a little olive oil over each bowl. Season with pepper, sprinkle with Parmesan cheese, and serve immediately. SERVES 6

sweet vidalia french onion soup

PROTEIN, HEALTHY FATS, VEGETABLES
DETOX, LEVEL 1, LEVEL 2

Slice the onions very thin with a sharp knife or a mandoline. Place a stockpot over medium-high heat. Add the 2 tablespoons olive oil and the onions. Sauté for about 10 minutes, then lower the heat to medium low. Add salt and pepper to taste, mustard seed, celery seed, and cracked peppercorns and continue to sauté the onions until caramelized to a deep golden brown, another 20 to 25 minutes.

When the onions are a rich brown, add the stock, wine, and Worcestershire. Turn the heat up to medium, and cook for about 15 minutes.

Preheat the broiler.

In the meantime, cut the stem off the portobello mushroom. Place the mushroom cap on its side and slice into 4 round thin pieces. Heat a large skillet over medium-high heat. Brush the mushroom slices with olive oil and place in the skillet, cooking for a couple of minutes on each side until lightly browned.

Ladle the soup into ovenproof bowls, preferably stoneware. Place a mushroom slice on top and then a slice of Gruyère. Put the bowls on a cookie sheet and place under the broiler for a minute or two, until the cheese gets brown and bubbly.   SERVES 4

NOTE Worcestershire sauce contains a small amount of sugar, but the small amount used creates only the slightest imbalance. If you are doing well on Level 1, feel free to add it.

3 sweet onions (Vidalia or Maui)

2 tablespoons olive oil, plus more for brushing

Sea salt and freshly ground black pepper

1 teaspoon mustard seed

1 teaspoon celery seed

1 teaspoon cracked black peppercorns

4 cups beef stock, preferably homemade (page 34)

$1/4$ cup dry red wine (omit for Detox)

1 tablespoon Worcestershire sauce (see Note; omit for Detox)

1 large portobello mushroom

4 slices Gruyère or provolone cheese

broccoli soup

2 tablespoons (¼ stick) unsalted butter

1 head broccoli, chopped

4 cups chicken stock or broth, preferably homemade (pages 30–32)

Sea salt and freshly ground black pepper

6 tablespoons sour cream (optional)

1 small bunch chives, chopped

Place a large stockpot over low heat. Add the butter and stir until just melted. Add the broccoli and sauté until tender, about 7 minutes. Add the chicken stock and bring to a boil. Lower the heat and simmer for 20 minutes.

Use a hand mixer to puree the broccoli in the pot. Leave the soup slightly chunky. If you do not have a hand mixer, take 2 cups of the mixture and puree in a food processor or blender. Add another 2 cups and partially puree, leaving the soup a little chunky. Add salt and pepper to taste.

Garnish with the sour cream, if using, sprinkle with the fresh chives, and serve immediately. SERVES 4 TO 6

broccoli leek soup

PROTEIN, HEALTHY FATS, VEGETABLES
DETOX, LEVEL 1, LEVEL 2

For the soup: Heat the olive oil in a stockpot. Add the leeks and sauté for about 5 minutes, until lightly browned. Add the stock and bring to a boil. Add the broccoli and bring back to a boil, then immediately reduce the heat and simmer for 15 minutes, until broccoli is soft. Season with salt and pepper. Use a hand mixer to puree the soup in the pot or transfer to a blender or food processor and blend until smooth.

For the garnish: Heat the olive oil in a skillet over medium heat, then add half the leeks and cook until golden brown. Remove with a slotted spoon and drain on paper towels. Repeat for the remaining leeks. Fry the garlic until golden brown; set aside with the leeks.

Ladle the soup into individual bowls and garnish each with a dollop of sour cream. Top with the fried leeks and garlic.   SERVES 6

SOUP
¼ cup olive oil

2 leeks, trimmed of dark green leaves, cleaned and chopped

8 cups chicken stock or broth, preferably homemade (pages 30–32)

6 cups chopped broccoli florets (about 3 stalks)

Sea salt and freshly ground black pepper

FRIED LEEK GARNISH
6 tablespoons olive oil

1 leek, trimmed of dark green leaves, cleaned and very thinly sliced

3 garlic cloves, finely chopped

6 tablespoons sour cream

cauliflower soup

PROTEIN, HEALTHY FATS, VEGETABLES

DETOX, LEVEL 1, LEVEL 2

2 tablespoons (¼ stick) unsalted butter

1 head cauliflower, chopped

4 cups chicken stock or broth, preferably homemade (pages 30–32)

Sea salt and freshly ground black pepper

6 tablespoons sour cream (optional)

1 small bunch chives, chopped

Place a stockpot over medium heat. Add the butter and stir until just melted. Add the cauliflower and sauté until tender, about 7 minutes. Add the stock and bring to a boil. Lower the heat and simmer for 20 minutes. Use a hand mixer to puree the cauliflower in the pot. Leave the soup slightly chunky. If you do not have a hand mixer, puree the mixture in a food processor or blender, keeping the soup a little chunky. Add salt and pepper to taste.

Garnish with the sour cream, if using, sprinkle with the chives, and serve immediately. SERVES 4 TO 6

red pepper soup with crispy sage leaves

PROTEIN, HEALTHY FATS, VEGETABLES

DETOX, LEVEL 1, LEVEL 2

For the soup: In a stockpot, combine the olive oil, celery, and onion. Cook over moderate heat until the vegetables are soft and fragrant, 10 to 15 minutes. And the red peppers and cook 3 to 4 minutes more. Season with salt. Add the celery root, 1 quart water, and the stock. Cover and cook over moderate heat until the celery root is soft, about 40 minutes.

For the garnish: Heat a medium skillet over medium heat. Pour in enough olive oil to cover bottom of pan. When the oil is hot but not smoking, add the sage leaves. Fry until crispy, 1 to 2 minutes. Drain on paper towels. Sprinkle with salt.

Puree the soup in the pot with a hand mixer or in batches in a blender or food processor. Ladle into warmed shallow soup bowls. Drizzle each bowl with crème fraîche in an attractive pattern. Sprinkle a few fried sage leaves on top and serve.   SERVES 6

SOUP

2 tablespoons olive oil

1 celery stalk, minced

1 onion, minced

6 Roasted Red Peppers (page 134), or jarred roasted peppers in water

Sea salt to taste

1 medium celery root, diced

2 cups chicken stock or broth, preferably homemade (pages 30–32)

FRIED SAGE LEAF GARNISH

Olive oil

40 fresh sage leaves, washed and patted dry

Sea salt

1/4 cup crème fraîche (page 149) or sour cream

roasted red pepper soup

3 cups vegetable stock, preferably homemade (page 33)

12 Roasted Red Peppers (page 134) or jarred roasted peppers in water

1 red onion, chopped

2 garlic cloves

1/4 teaspoon red pepper flakes

Sea salt and freshly ground black pepper

1/4 cup chopped fresh cilantro

In a stockpot, bring the stock to a boil. Add the red peppers, onion, garlic, and red pepper flakes. Bring back to a boil, then immediately reduce the heat and simmer for about 10 minutes.

Use a hand mixer to puree the soup in the pot or transfer to a blender or food processor and blend until smooth. Add salt and pepper to taste. Ladle into bowls and garnish with cilantro.   SERVES 6

roasted tomato soup

PROTEIN, HEALTHY FATS, VEGETABLES

LEVEL 1, LEVEL 2

Preheat the oven to 350°F.

Cut the tomatoes in half through the middle and lay them cut side up on a baking sheet or roasting pan. Drizzle olive oil on top of the tomatoes. Sprinkle the tomatoes liberally with sea salt. Top with the thyme leaves or seasoning rub. Place the tomatoes into the oven for about 2 hours, or until slightly darkened on top.

When done, remove from the oven and scrape into a medium saucepan, including the drippings from the bottom of the baking sheet. Add the chopped basil. Bring to a boil over medium heat for 10 minutes. Then add the chicken stock, reduce the heat, and simmer for 45 minutes. Add the All Natural SomerSweet and red pepper flakes, if using. Remove from the heat and puree the soup in the pot with a hand mixer or transfer to a blender or food processor and puree until smooth. Stir in the heavy cream and adjust the seasoning. Ladle into serving bowls, garnish with a dollop of sour cream, and sprinkle with julienned basil.

SERVES 4 TO 6

10 ripe tomatoes

$1/4$ cup olive oil

Sea salt and freshly ground black pepper

1 bunch fresh thyme, leaves only, or 1 tablespoon Somersize Tuscan Sea Salt Rub

1 bunch fresh basil, coarsely chopped, plus 10 whole leaves, julienned, for garnish

2 cups chicken stock or broth, preferably homemade (pages 30–32)

2 teaspoons All Natural SomerSweet (or more to taste)

$1/8$ teaspoon red pepper flakes (optional)

$1/4$ cup heavy cream

Sour cream or crème fraîche (page 149), for garnish

watercress mushroom soup

PROTEIN, HEALTHY FATS, VEGETABLES

DETOX, LEVEL 1, LEVEL 2

3 tablespoons unsalted butter

8 ounces white mushrooms, chopped

1 large onion, chopped

2 bunches watercress, chopped

2 garlic cloves, chopped

4 cups chicken stock or broth, preferably homemade (pages 30–32)

Sea salt and freshly ground black pepper

5 tablespoons heavy cream

Heat a large sauté pan over medium heat and add the butter. When butter is melted, add the mushrooms and onion. Sauté about 5 minutes. Add the watercress and garlic, and sauté for another 10 minutes. Stir in 2 cups of stock.

Puree the mixture in the pot using a hand mixer or transfer to a blender or food processor.

Return the mixture to a saucepan and add rest of the stock. Season to taste with salt and pepper. Stir in the cream just before serving. SERVES 4 TO 6

mushroom lemon soup

PROTEIN, HEALTHY FATS, VEGETABLES

DETOX, LEVEL 1, LEVEL 2

2 onions, quartered

1 pound fresh shiitake mushrooms

3 tablespoons olive oil

6 cups chicken stock or broth, preferably homemade (pages 30–32)

Sea salt and freshly ground black pepper

4 lemons, 3 halved and 1 thinly sliced

Puree the onions in a food processor.

Clean the mushrooms by gently dusting with a mushroom brush, then finely chop in a food processor.

In a medium saucepan, heat the olive oil. Cook the onions in the saucepan until translucent, then add the mushrooms and cook for 10 minutes. Add the stock and salt and pepper to taste, and simmer for 30 minutes.

Ladle the soup into bowls and squeeze the juice from ½ lemon into each bowl. Garnish each bowl with a lemon slice. SERVES 6

pumpkin soup with roasted shallots and sage

PROTEIN, HEALTHY FATS, VEGETABLES, INSULIN TRIGGERS

LEVEL 2

Preheat the oven to 350°F.

Quarter and seed the pumpkin if using fresh. Rub the flesh with the 4 tablespoons olive oil and bake on a baking sheet for 30 minutes. Set aside to cool.

Melt 4 tablespoons of butter in a stockpot over medium heat. Cook the onions in the butter until translucent, about 7 minutes. Add the garlic and cook 1 minute longer. Meanwhile, scrape the flesh from the pumpkin (or use canned pumpkin) and add to the onions. Cook for about 5 minutes.

Add 4 cups of the stock to the pot and simmer for 30 minutes. Use a hand mixer to puree the soup in the pot. Otherwise, transfer the soup to a blender or food processor and puree until smooth, then return it to the pot. If necessary, thin the soup with the remaining stock. Season to taste with salt and pepper. Set the soup aside and keep it warm.

Melt the remaining 2 tablespoons butter in a small pan over medium heat and cook the shallots until golden and tender, about 15 minutes.

Heat the 1 cup olive oil in a deep pot over medium heat. Add the sage leaves and fry until crisp, 1 to 2 minutes. Drain on paper towels. Garnish each serving with 3 shallot halves and 3 sage leaves.

SERVES 4 TO 6

1 small pumpkin, about 5 pounds, or two 29-ounce cans pumpkin (not pie mix)

4 tablespoons plus 1 cup olive oil

6 tablespoons (³/4 stick) unsalted butter

2 medium onions, finely chopped ·

2 garlic cloves, peeled and minced

4 to 6 cups chicken stock or broth, preferably homemade (pages 30–32)

Sea salt and freshly ground black pepper

9 shallots, peeled and halved lengthwise

20 fresh sage leaves

split pea soup

1 pound dried split peas, rinsed

8 cups vegetable stock, preferably homemade (page 33)

2 cups chopped onions

2 tablespoons fresh dill

2 dried bay leaves

Sea salt and freshly ground black pepper

Nonfat sour cream or yogurt, for garnish

Soak the split peas according to package directions. In a stockpot, bring 1 cup of the stock to a boil. Add the onions, lower the heat, and simmer until the onions are soft, about 5 minutes. Add the rest of the stock, the split peas, dill, and bay leaves. Bring to a boil, reduce the heat, and simmer, covered, for 1½ hours, or until split peas are tender. Remove bay leaves. Season with salt and pepper, garnish with nonfat sour cream or yogurt, and serve.

The soup may also be pureed before serving, for a smooth consistency.   SERVES 8

tex-mex black bean soup

VEGETABLES, CARBOHYDRATES

DETOX, LEVEL 1, LEVEL 2

In a medium saucepan over medium-high heat, bring 1 cup of the stock to a boil. Add the onion and cook in the stock for 6 minutes. Add the beans, remaining stock, the cumin, Tabasco, and cayenne. Simmer for 5 minutes. Puree the soup with a hand mixer or transfer to a food processor and puree for 30 seconds. Season with salt and pepper. Add the cilantro and lime juice, and stir well. Serve immediately, with a dollop of fresh salsa. SERVES 4

4 cups vegetable stock, preferably homemade (page 33)

1 cup chopped onion

Three 15-ounce cans fat-free black beans, drained

1 tablespoon plus 2 teaspoons ground cumin

1 teaspoon Tabasco sauce

1/4 teaspoon cayenne

Sea salt and freshly ground black pepper

3 tablespoons chopped fresh cilantro

2 tablespoons fresh lime juice

Salsa, for garnish

lentil soup

1 pound lentils

6 cups vegetable
stock, preferably
homemade
(page 33), or water

2 slices fresh ginger

1 medium onion,
chopped

Sea salt and freshly
ground black pepper

2 bunches cilantro,
stemmed and
chopped

5 or 6 lemons

1 bunch basil, stemmed
and chopped

Lemon slices, for
garnish

Place the lentils in a stockpot. Add the stock, ginger, and onion. Bring to a boil, reduce the heat, and simmer for about 90 minutes, or until the lentils are tender.

Use a hand mixer to puree the soup in the pot or transfer to a blender or food processor and puree for 30 seconds. Add the salt, pepper, and cilantro.

Ladle the soup into bowls and squeeze the juice of ½ lemon into each bowl. Garnish with liberal amounts of the basil and a thin slice of lemon.   SERVES 10 TO 12

red lentil cumin soup

PROTEIN, VEGETABLES, CARBOHYDRATES

DETOX, LEVEL 1, LEVEL 2

In a large pot, bring ½ cup of the stock to a boil. Add the onion, reduce the heat, and simmer until onion is soft and most of the liquid has evaporated. Add the ginger, garlic, cumin, and tomatoes. Stir to combine. Simmer over low heat for 2 minutes.

Add the lentils and the remaining 4½ cups stock. Bring to a boil, reduce the heat, and simmer for 20 to 25 minutes. Season to taste with salt and pepper. Garnish with the scallions. SERVES 6

5 cups chicken stock or broth, preferably homemade (pages 30–32)

1 medium onion, chopped

¼ teaspoon crushed fresh ginger

¼ teaspoon pressed garlic

1 teaspoon ground cumin

One 14-ounce can crushed tomatoes

3 cups (1 pound) red lentils, rinsed

Sea salt and freshly ground black pepper

4 scallions, white and green parts, sliced

cold cucumber-asparagus soup

VEGETABLES, CARBOHYDRATES

DETOX, LEVEL 1, LEVEL 2

1½ cups chopped asparagus (about 35 stalks), tough ends removed

2 cups vegetable stock, preferably homemade (page 33)

2 medium cucumbers, peeled, seeded, and chopped

1 tablespoon finely chopped fresh dill

Sea salt and freshly ground black pepper

4 tablespoons plain nonfat yogurt

4 sprigs fresh dill

Place about 2 cups of water in the bottom of a pan fitted with a steaming basket and a lid. Heat on high until the water boils. Put the asparagus in the steamer, cover, and cook until tender, approximately 4 minutes. Remove the asparagus and rinse under cool water. Transfer the cooled asparagus to a blender or food processor. Add the stock, cucumbers, and dill. Blend until smooth. Puree in two batches if necessary.

Season the soup to taste with salt and pepper. Chill in the refrigerator for at least 1 hour, then serve with a dollop of yogurt and a sprig of fresh dill.   SERVES 4

salads
beyond greens

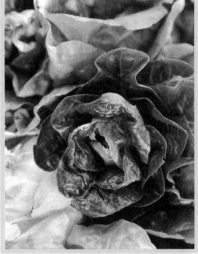

One of the great joys in my life is walking to my organic vegetable garden each day when we are at our home in the desert and picking the outer leaves of my beautiful variety of lettuces for the perfect salad. At the beach I don't have the room for a big garden, but I get an incredible yield from growing lettuce in a small pot. I call it my pot garden! We still have more than we can eat, with leftovers to share.

With nature's perfectly grown starter, all you need is a good bottle of olive oil, fresh lemons, and an excellent-quality sea salt. These simple ingredients, to me, make the ultimate salad. From there, the variations and possibilities are endless! For entrée salads, I add everything from protein and vegetables to cheeses and nuts. We've come a long way from my childhood when salad was iceberg lettuce with a lousy bottled Thousand Island dressing.

If you are a lover of classics, in this section you'll enjoy the Caesar (page 86), Cobb (page 85), and Greek (page 78) salads, and the Southern Country Fried Chicken Salad (page 94) with Green Goddess Dressing (page 146). If you are a foodie, explore exciting creations like the Chopped Raw Zucchini and Parmesan Salad (also known as "what to do when zucchini is growing like crazy," page 63), Spicy Rock Shrimp Salad (buttery little shrimp with a fresh POW! of taste from chiles and lime, page 82), Baby Artichoke Salad (with shaved tender baby artichokes, yum, page 77). And make sure to try my twice-a-week staple, the Israeli Salad with finely chopped tomatoes, radishes, peppers, and cucumbers (page 74). Salads are a lovely, fresh and delicious way to stock up on nutrition.

blue cheese vinaigrette with crudités

PROTEIN, HEALTHY FATS, VEGETABLES

DETOX, LEVEL 1, LEVEL 2

Cut the zucchini, cucumber, peppers, and celery into strips of equal length, about 5 inches. Arrange all the prepared vegetables on a platter with the vinaigrette in a small bowl in the center.　SERVES 8

2 medium zucchini

1 hothouse cucumber

1 yellow bell pepper, seeded

1 red bell pepper, seeded

5 celery stalks

$^1/_2$ pound fresh snow peas

10 asparagus stalks, blanched (see page 159)

Blue Cheese Vinaigrette (page 145)

arugula and parmesan salad

PROTEIN, HEALTHY FATS, VEGETABLES, CARBOHYDRATES

LEVEL 1, LEVEL 2

Preheat the oven to 350°F.

Spread the nuts loosely on a baking sheet. Toast until lightly browned, 8 to 10 minutes. Check every few minutes to avoid burning the nuts. Remove from the oven and turn out onto a large plate to cool. (The nuts can be toasted several hours in advance.)

In a large, shallow salad bowl, combine the arugula and toasted pine nuts. Using a vegetable peeler, shave the Parmesan cheese into long, thick strips directly into the bowl. (When the wedge of cheese becomes too small to peel, grate the remaining cheese and add it to the bowl.)

Drizzle the olive oil and vinegar over the salad and toss. Season to taste with salt and pepper. Serve immediately.　SERVES 4

$^1/_2$ cup pine nuts

1 pound arugula leaves, stems removed, or baby spinach leaves

A 2-ounce wedge Parmesan cheese

About 4 tablespoons extra virgin olive oil

About 2 tablespoons red wine vinegar

Sea salt and freshly ground black pepper

garden greens with pear tomatoes and lemon-mint vinaigrette

HEALTHY FATS, VEGETABLES

DETOX, LEVEL 1, LEVEL 2

LEMON-MINT VINAIGRETTE

¼ cup white wine vinegar

1 tablespoon chopped fresh mint leaves

Sea salt and freshly ground black pepper

½ cup extra virgin olive oil

SALAD

½ head red leaf lettuce

1 head butter lettuce

1 small head frisée (curly baby endive)

1 pint yellow pear or cherry tomatoes

Zest of 1 lemon

For the vinaigrette: Whisk together the vinegar, mint leaves, and salt and pepper to taste in a mixing cup. Add the oil in a slow stream, whisking constantly until the oil is emulsified.

For the salad: Wash and dry the lettuces and tear them into bite-size pieces. Combine with the tomatoes in a large salad bowl.

Toss the salad with the vinaigrette. Garnish with the lemon zest and serve immediately.   SERVES 6

iceberg wedge with roquefort dressing

HEALTHY FATS, VEGETABLES

DETOX, LEVEL 1, LEVEL 2

ROQUEFORT DRESSING

4 ounces crumbled blue cheese, preferably Roquefort

¾ cup sour cream

1 tablespoon red wine vinegar

Sea salt and freshly ground black pepper

1 head iceberg lettuce

1 pint cherry tomatoes

Combine the dressing ingredients in a food processor and blend until well mixed, or blend the ingredients in a bowl with a whisk. If the dressing is too thick for your liking, add more vinegar until you reach the desired consistency. (Makes 1½ cups.)

Cut the lettuce into 6 large wedges and place on serving plates. Add a generous amount of roquefort dressing and cracked black pepper. Garnish with tomatoes.   SERVES 6

chopped raw zucchini and parmesan salad

HEALTHY FATS, VEGETABLES

DETOX, LEVEL 1, LEVEL 2

Trim the ends off the zucchini. Slice into ¼-inch pieces, then coarsely chop into bite-size pieces and set aside.

Wash and dry the lettuce leaves, discarding any imperfect ones.

In a salad bowl, whisk together the olive oil, lemon juice, and salt and pepper to taste until well combined. Add the zucchini and toss until well coated.

Using a sharp knife or cheese shaver, cut long, paper-thin slices of Parmesan. Place over the top of the zucchini.

Divide the lettuce among six serving plates. Spoon the chopped and seasoned zucchini on top of the lettuce. Garnish with a few extra shavings of Parmesan. Season with additional salt and pepper and serve immediately. SERVES 6

2 pounds slender zucchini (up to 1 ½ inches in diameter)

1 pound Boston lettuce

3 to 4 tablespoons extra virgin olive oil

2 tablespoons fresh lemon juice, or more to taste

Sea salt and freshly ground black pepper

A 4-ounce wedge Parmesan cheese

zucchini carpaccio

3 medium zucchini

3 bunches arugula

$^1/_3$ cup extra virgin olive oil

2 lemons

Sea salt and freshly ground black pepper

Shavings of Parmesan cheese

HEALTHY FATS, VEGETABLES

DETOX, LEVEL 1, LEVEL 2

Slice the zucchini lengthwise as thin as possible using a mandoline or vegetable peeler. Rinse and dry the arugula and place into a bowl. Drizzle a little of the olive oil over the arugula, then squeeze the juice of 1 lemon on top. Toss with salt and pepper. Arrange the arugula on six plates.

Place the raw zucchini slices in a single layer over the arugula to cover it completely. Drizzle the zucchini with a little more olive oil and the juice from the remaining lemon. Sprinkle with salt and pepper, then top with Parmesan cheese.   SERVES 6

tricolore salad with balsamic vinaigrette

1 pound mixed lettuces (radicchio, arugula, endive), rinsed and dried

Balsamic Vinaigrette (page 143)

Sea salt and freshly ground black pepper

HEALTHY FATS, VEGETABLES

DETOX, LEVEL 1, LEVEL 2

Tear the lettuces into bite-size pieces and place in a large bowl. Toss with the vinaigrette just before serving. Season to taste with salt and pepper.   SERVES 8

baby greens with champagne vinaigrette

HEALTHY FATS, VEGETABLES

DETOX, LEVEL 1, LEVEL 2

Place the vinegar in a mixing cup with the basil and salt and pepper to taste. Add the olive oil in a slow stream, constantly whisking until the oil is emulsified.

In a large bowl toss the washed greens with the vinaigrette. Garnish each serving with a sprinkle of pomegranate seeds, if using.   SERVES 8

2 tablespoons Champagne vinegar

1 teaspoon finely chopped fresh basil leaves

Sea salt and freshly ground black pepper

6 tablespoons extra virgin olive oil

1 pound mixed baby greens, washed

1/3 cup pomegranate seeds (for Level 2 only)

green salad with artichoke hearts and red wine vinaigrette

HEALTHY FATS, VEGETABLES

DETOX, LEVEL 1, LEVEL 2

   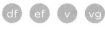

Tear the lettuces into bite-size pieces and place in a large bowl. Toss with the artichoke hearts, onion, and vinaigrette. Season to taste with salt and pepper. Serve immediately.   SERVES 4

1 pound mixed lettuces (red leaf, butter, romaine), rinsed and dried

One 8-ounce jar marinated artichoke hearts, drained

1/2 medium red onion, chopped

Red Wine Vinaigrette (page 143)

Sea salt and freshly ground black pepper

spinach salad with hot bacon dressing

PROTEIN, HEALTHY FATS, VEGETABLES

DETOX, LEVEL 1, LEVEL 2

$^{1}/_{2}$ pound bacon, cut
into 1-inch pieces

3 tablespoons balsamic
vinegar

$^{1}/_{2}$ pound fresh spinach
leaves, washed and
dried thoroughly

Sea salt and freshly
ground black pepper

2 large hard-boiled
eggs, peeled and
chopped

10 cherry tomatoes

Place a large skillet over medium heat. Add the bacon and fry until golden brown, stirring with a wooden spoon to separate the pieces. (If the bacon is burning on the edges, lower the heat.) Turn off the heat, then immediately remove the bacon and drain on paper towels.

Pour off all but 2 tablespoons of bacon fat from the hot skillet. Place the skillet back on the stove over medium-high heat. Add the balsamic vinegar and heat for approximately 1 minute while scraping all the bits from the bottom of the skillet.

Place the spinach in a salad bowl. Pour on the hot bacon dressing and toss. Season with salt and pepper. Divide the salad between two plates. Crumble the fried bacon and sprinkle over the salads. Sprinkle on the chopped hard-boiled eggs and garnish with cherry tomatoes. SERVES 2

buffalo mozzarella and cherry tomato salad

HEALTHY FATS, VEGETABLES

DETOX, LEVEL 1, LEVEL 2

Cut the tomatoes in half and place in a large salad bowl. Cut the mozzarella into chunks roughly the size of the cherry tomato halves, then add to the salad bowl. Julienne the basil leaves and add to the tomatoes and mozzarella. Drizzle the olive oil over the top, then season with salt and a liberal amount of coarsely ground pepper. Toss and serve.   SERVES 4

2 pints cherry tomatoes

One 8-ounce ball buffalo mozzarella

1 bunch fresh basil, stemmed

2 tablespoons extra virgin olive oil

Sea salt and freshly ground black pepper

buffalo mozzarella, fennel, and celery salad

HEALTHY FATS, VEGETABLES

DETOX, LEVEL 1, LEVEL 2

Place the fennel, celery, and mozzarella in a large salad bowl. Toss with the lemon juice, olive oil, and salt and pepper to taste. Serve immediately.   SERVES 4

1 fennel bulb, trimmed and chopped

4 celery stalks, chopped

One 8-ounce ball buffalo mozzarella, chopped into bite-size pieces

Juice of 1 lemon

$1/4$ cup extra virgin olive oil

Sea salt and freshly ground black pepper

tomato and cucumber salad with feta vinaigrette

HEALTHY FATS, VEGETABLES
DETOX, LEVEL 1, LEVEL 2

1 tablespoon balsamic
vinegar

¼ teaspoon sea salt

¼ teaspoon coarsely
ground black pepper

¼ cup extra virgin olive
oil

6 ounces crumbled feta
cheese

4 Roma (plum)
tomatoes, sliced

1 small English
cucumber, sliced

½ cup Kalamata olives
(for Level 1 and
Level 2)

Place the balsamic vinegar in a small bowl. Add salt and pepper. Whisk in the olive oil a little at a time until oil emulsifies and vinaigrette is creamy. Stir in feta cheese. Cover and refrigerate until ready to use.

To serve, place slices of tomato and cucumber on individual salad plates. Drizzle with the vinaigrette, being sure to spoon some of the feta on top of each. Garnish with olives, if using.   SERVES 6

endive and radicchio salad with stilton cheese

HEALTHY FATS, VEGETABLES
DETOX, LEVEL 1, LEVEL 2

3 heads radicchio,
leaves separated

3 Belgian endive, leaves
separated

8 ounces Stilton cheese,
crumbled

Balsamic Vinaigrette
(page 143)

1 cup toasted walnuts
(for Level 1 and
Level 2)

Arrange 3 radicchio leaves on each serving plate. Fan 4 or 5 endive leaves in a pretty pattern. Crumble the Stilton on top.

Drizzle the vinaigrette over the salads. Garnish with walnuts, if using.   SERVES 8

maytag blue cheese and roasted vegetable salad

PROTEIN, HEALTHY FATS, VEGETABLES

DETOX, LEVEL 1, LEVEL 2

Preheat the oven to 350°F.

Rub a 9 × 12-inch baking dish with 1 tablespoon of the olive oil. Cut the onion and garlic in half (around the equator or the middle) and drizzle each half with the remaining olive oil. Place the onion, garlic, peppers, and tomatoes in the pan. Reduce the heat to 300°F and roast the vegetables for 1 hour, until vegetables are browned.

Remove the baking dish from the oven. Quickly cover with a baking sheet to "steam" the vegetables, setting them aside for 15 minutes. Peel the skin off and remove the seeds from the peppers and tomatoes.

Toss the lettuce with the vinaigrette. Arrange on four large salad plates. Slice the onion and divide among the salads. Coarsely chop the peppers and tomatoes, and divide among the salads. Squeeze the roasted garlic cloves from their skins (at least 3 cloves per salad) and spread over the peppers and onion. Divide the cheese and crumble over each salad. Pour a little of the juice from the bottom of the baking pan over the cheese, and serve. SERVES 4

2 tablespoons olive oil

1 medium Bermuda onion

1 head garlic

1 large yellow bell pepper

1 large red bell pepper

2 ripe medium tomatoes

2 heads Bibb lettuce (about 1 pound), washed, dried, and torn into pieces

$^3/_4$ cup Herb Vinaigrette (page 144)

4 ounces crumbled Maytag blue cheese

lamb's lettuce salad with warmed goat cheese

HEALTHY FATS, VEGETABLES

DETOX, LEVEL 1, LEVEL 2

1 cup extra virgin olive oil

2 garlic cloves, crushed

Sea salt and freshly ground black pepper

12 fresh basil leaves

Twelve 1-inch-thick slices mild goat cheese

1/2 cup freshly grated Romano cheese

1 pound mâche

3/4 cup Herb Vinaigrette (page 144)

In a mixing cup, combine the oil, garlic, salt and pepper to taste, and basil. Place the goat cheese in a shallow dish and pour the oil over it. Let marinate for at least 1 hour, basting frequently.

Preheat the oven to 450°F. Remove the cheese from the oil, reserving the oil for the vinaigrette. Coat the goat cheese with the grated romano on both sides and place on a baking sheet. Bake for 6 to 10 minutes, until the cheese begins to bubble.

Toss the mâche with the vinaigrette and arrange on six plates. Place 2 slices of warmed goat cheese on each plate and serve immediately. SERVES 6

chanterelle salad with creamy parmesan dressing

PROTEIN, HEALTHY FATS, VEGETABLES

DETOX, LEVEL 1, LEVEL 2

For the salad: Combine the arugula, endive, tomato, and onion in a large salad bowl.

Place a skillet over medium-high heat and add the olive oil. Sauté the chanterelle mushrooms for 5 to 7 minutes. Remove from the heat and set aside to cool.

For the dressing: Bring a small saucepan of water to a boil. Add the egg and cook for 30 seconds. Remove with a slotted spoon to cool. When cool enough to touch, crack the egg and place the yolk in a mixing bowl. Discard the white. Add all the remaining dressing ingredients except the oil and Parmesan. Whisk until well combined. Then add the oil and 1½ tablespoons warm water, and whisk until emulsified. Last, stir in the grated cheese.

Add the mushrooms to the salad bowl and toss the salad with the dressing. Garnish with shaved Parmesan cheese. Serve immediately. SERVES 4

SALAD

1/2 pound arugula

3 Belgian endive, chopped

1 Roma (plum) tomato, chopped

1/2 red onion, thinly sliced

1 tablespoon olive oil

3 ounces fresh chanterelle mushrooms

Shavings of Parmesan cheese

CREAMY PARMESAN DRESSING

1 large egg

1/2 tablespoons mayonnaise

1 tablespoon Dijon mustard

1 tablespoon anchovy paste (optional)

1 tablespoon minced garlic

1 tablespoon Worcestershire sauce (see Note, page 45)

1 tablespoon red wine vinegar

1 teaspoon hot pepper sauce

1/2 tablespoons fresh lemon juice

Sea salt and freshly ground black pepper

1/2 teaspoons extra virgin olive oil

3 tablespoons freshly grated Parmesan cheese

baby spinach salad with vidalia onions, sun-dried tomatoes, and goat cheese

PROTEIN, HEALTHY FATS, VEGETABLES

DETOX, LEVEL 1, LEVEL 2

8 strips lean bacon

5 tablespoons extra virgin olive oil

1 large Vidalia onion, thinly sliced

1 teaspoon crushed garlic

¼ cup balsamic vinegar

1 teaspoon sea salt

1 teaspoon freshly ground black pepper

¾ cup chopped sun-dried tomatoes

1 pound fresh baby spinach

10 to 12 ounces goat cheese, sliced into 8 rounds

Cut the bacon strips into 1-inch pieces. Heat a large skillet over medium-high heat. Add 2 tablespoons of the olive oil and heat for a minute or two. Add the bacon and fry until golden brown, gently separating the pieces by stirring with a wooden spoon. Remove the bacon and drain on paper towels.

Pour off all the bacon fat from skillet. Place skillet back on the stove over medium heat, and add the onion (with a little olive oil, if necessary). Sauté the onion for approximately 10 minutes, until golden brown and beginning to caramelize. Add the garlic and cook for 1 minute.

Stir the vinegar, salt, and pepper into the onion mixture, scraping the pan to get the browned bits off the bottom. Add the sun-dried tomatoes and remaining 3 tablespoons olive oil, stirring constantly to blend the flavors.

Divide the spinach among four large salad plates. Place 2 thick rounds of goat cheese on each salad. Sprinkle the bacon pieces on top of the cheese, then place the warm onion-tomato mixture over the salad. Drizzle the hot dressing over the cheese and spinach. SERVES 4

hearts of palm and artichoke salad

HEALTHY FATS, VEGETABLES

DETOX, LEVEL 1, LEVEL 2

Combine the hearts of palm, celery, artichoke hearts, and parsley in a large salad bowl. Toss with the vinaigrette. Season to taste with salt and pepper and serve. SERVES 4

One 14-ounce can hearts of palm, drained and chopped

6 celery stalks, chopped

Two 6^1/2-ounce jars marinated artichoke hearts, drained

1 bunch flat-leaf parsley, chopped

1 cup Red Wine Vinaigrette (page 143)

Sea salt and freshly ground black pepper

fennel, red onion, and hearts of palm salad

HEALTHY FATS, VEGETABLES

DETOX, LEVEL 1, LEVEL 2

Trim the stalks from the fennel and thinly slice the fennel bulb. Place fennel in a large salad bowl and add the onion. Carefully cut the hearts of palm into ¼-inch slices and add to bowl. Chop the basil leaves coarsely and add, then season with salt and pepper. Add the dressing to the salad and toss gently, taking care not to break the hearts of palm. Refrigerate for 1 hour before serving. SERVES 4

2 large fennel bulbs

1 medium red or other sweet onion, thinly sliced

One 14-ounce can hearts of palm, drained

^{1}/4 cup packed fresh basil leaves

Sea salt and freshly ground black pepper

^{2}/3 cup Pink Goddess Salad Dressing (page 147)

green bean salad and hearts of palm

HEALTHY FATS, VEGETABLES

DETOX, LEVEL 1, LEVEL 2

Sea salt

1 pound green beans

One 14-ounce can
hearts of palm,
drained

2 Roma (plum)
tomatoes, seeded
and chopped

2 small red onions,
thinly sliced

1 bunch flat-leaf parsley,
chopped

2 ounces crumbled feta
cheese

1 cup Red Wine
Vinaigrette
(page 143)

Freshly ground black
pepper

Bring a medium saucepan of salted water to a boil. Add the beans and boil 3 to 4 minutes, until tender. The beans will change from light to dark green. Drain and plunge the beans into a bowl of ice water; the ice bath stops the cooking process, sets the flavor, and helps the beans retain their dark green color. Slice the blanched green beans on the diagonal into 1-inch pieces and place in a large salad bowl.

Slice the hearts of palm on the diagonal into 1-inch pieces. Add the hearts of palm, tomatoes, onions, parsley, and feta to the bowl. Toss with the vinaigrette and season with additional salt and pepper.   SERVES 4

israeli salad

HEALTHY FATS, VEGETABLES

DETOX, LEVEL 1, LEVEL 2

6 or 7 Kirby or Persian
cucumbers, or
1 regular cucumber,
seeded

4 or 5 tomatoes,
seeded

1 green bell pepper,
cored and seeded

3 scallions, trimmed

4 radishes

Sea salt and freshly
ground black pepper

Extra virgin olive oil

Lemon wedges

Finely dice all the vegetables into a uniform size. Toss with salt and pepper. Serve immediately with a drizzle of olive oil and a wedge of lemon.   SERVES 6

jícama and snap pea citrus salad

HEALTHY FATS, VEGETABLES

DETOX, LEVEL 1, LEVEL 2

Marinate the onion in the lime juice with a little salt and let stand for a few hours.

Combine the jícama and sugar snap peas. Toss with the vinaigrette. Place on individual salad plates and garnish each with a handful of the marinated onion.   SERVES 4

1 red onion, sliced
  paper-thin

Juice of 6 limes

Sea salt

2 cups peeled and
  julienned jícama

2 cups sugar snap peas,
  julienned

3/4 cup Lemon-Mint
  Vinaigrette
  (page 62)

crunchy cabbage salad

HEALTHY FATS, VEGETABLES

DETOX, LEVEL 1, LEVEL 2

Combine all the ingredients in a large salad bowl. Refrigerate for at least 1 hour to let the flavors combine. Season to taste with salt and pepper and serve.   SERVES 6

1/2 head green cabbage,
  shredded

1/2 head red cabbage,
  shredded

1 bunch flat-leaf parsley,
  chopped

1 medium red onion,
  thinly sliced

1 cup Red Wine
  Vinaigrette
  (page 143)

Sea salt and freshly
  ground black pepper

crunchy coleslaw

1 fennel bulb, trimmed
and thinly sliced

2 cups shredded green
cabbage

2 cups shredded red
cabbage

3 scallions, white and
green parts, thinly
sliced

$1/2$ cup mayonnaise

$1/2$ cup sour cream

2 teaspoons lemon juice

1 teaspoon All Natural
SomerSweet

$1/8$ teaspoon Tabasco
sauce

1 teaspoon apple cider
vinegar

1 teaspoon celery seed
(optional)

Sea salt and freshly
ground black pepper

Place the fennel, green and red cabbage, and scallions in a large mixing bowl. In a separate small bowl, stir together the mayonnaise, sour cream, lemon juice, All Natural SomerSweet, Tabasco, and vinegar. Season with the celery seed, if desired, and salt and pepper. Toss the dressing and vegetables. Refrigerate until ready to serve. SERVES 4

baby artichoke salad

HEALTHY FATS, VEGETABLES

DETOX, LEVEL 1, LEVEL 2

24 baby artichokes

6 lemons

5 tablespoons extra
virgin olive oil

1/4 cup chopped flat-
leaf parsley, plus
4 sprigs for garnish

Sea salt and freshly
ground black pepper

1/2 cup thin shavings of
Parmesan cheese

Trim the bottoms and remove the tough outer green leaves from the artichokes until all that remains are the hearts with the yellowish tender leaves attached. Wash and rub with the cut side of 1 lemon to prevent discoloration. Keep the artichokes in water with the juice from 1 lemon until ready to slice.

Slice the artichokes lengthwise *very thin* (a mandoline is helpful). Toss with the olive oil, juice from 3 lemons, the parsley, salt, and pepper. Arrange on four plates and top with generous amounts of cheese shavings. Cut the remaining lemon into quarters and garnish each plate with a lemon wedge and a sprig of parsley.   SERVES 4

baby greens with sherry shallot vinaigrette

HEALTHY FATS, VEGETABLES

DETOX, LEVEL 1, LEVEL 2

1/2 pound mixed baby
greens

1/4 cup sherry vinegar

2 tablespoons finely
minced shallots

Sea salt and freshly
ground black pepper

3/4 cup extra virgin
olive oil

Wash the greens and set aside. In a mixing bowl, combine the vinegar shallots, and salt and pepper to taste. Slowly add the oil in a steady stream, whisking until emulsified. Toss the greens in the vinaigrette until coated. Serve immediately.   SERVES 2

greek salad

HEALTHY FATS, VEGETABLES
DETOX, LEVEL 1, LEVEL 2

3 ripe medium tomatoes, chopped

1 medium cucumber, chopped

8 ounces crumbled feta cheese

1/2 red onion, chopped

3 tablespoons extra virgin olive oil

Juice from 1/2 lemon

Freshly ground black pepper

Pinch of dried oregano

Couple sprigs of fresh basil

Kalamata olives (for Level 1 and Level 2)

Combine the tomatoes, cucumber, feta cheese, and red onion in a medium bowl. Mix, then drizzle with olive oil and lemon juice. Grind the black pepper over the top of the salad, sprinkle with a touch of oregano, and garnish with basil sprigs and olives, if using. Adjust seasoning to taste. SERVES 4

asian greens with soy vinaigrette

HEALTHY FATS, VEGETABLES
DETOX, LEVEL 1, LEVEL 2

1/2 pound mixed baby greens, preferably baby Asian (mizuna, tatsoi, mustard)

1 tablespoon soy sauce

1/4 cup extra virgin olive oil

3/4 cup olive oil

Sea salt and freshly ground black pepper

Juice from 1/4 lime

Wash the greens and set aside. Combine the remaining ingredients in a salad bowl. Add the greens and toss to coat. Serve immediately. SERVES 2

broccoli and cauliflower with lemon-garlic vinaigrette

HEALTHY FATS, VEGETABLES

DETOX, LEVEL 1, LEVEL 2

1 bunch broccoli

1 medium cauliflower

LEMON-GARLIC
  VINAIGRETTE

2 tablespoons fresh
  lemon juice, or more
  as desired

2 garlic cloves, pressed

Sea salt and freshly
  ground black pepper

6 tablespoons extra
  virgin olive oil

Wash the broccoli and cauliflower. Trim the tough ends off the stalks. Chop the remaining broccoli and cauliflower into large pieces. Put water in the bottom of a large pot fitted with a steamer over high heat. Add the broccoli and cauliflower, and steam until tender, 10 to 12 minutes.

For the vinaigrette: Place the lemon juice, garlic, and salt and pepper to taste in a mixing cup. Add the olive oil in a slow stream, constantly whisking until the oil is emulsified. For a tangier dressing, add more lemon juice.

Toss the broccoli and cauliflower in the vinaigrette and serve immediately.   SERVES 6

artichoke bottoms with dungeness crab salad

PROTEIN, HEALTHY FATS, VEGETABLES
DETOX, LEVEL 1, LEVEL 2

¹/₂ pound fresh Dungeness crabmeat

¹/₄ cup finely diced celery

¹/₄ cup finely diced onion

Juice from ¹/₂ lemon

¹/₄ cup mayonnaise

Sea salt and freshly ground black pepper

8 artichoke bottoms, freshly steamed or canned in water

Chopped flat-leaf parsley, for garnish

Pick through the crabmeat to remove any shells. Place into a large mixing bowl and add all the ingredients except the artichokes and parsley. Stir to combine and season with salt and pepper. Fill each artichoke bottom with the crab mixture. Garnish with the parsley and serve immediately. SERVES 8

apple salad with blue cheese vinaigrette

HEALTHY FATS, VEGETABLES, FRUIT
LEVEL 2

¹/₄ cup crumbled blue cheese

¹/₄ cup sherry vinegar

³/₄ cup extra virgin olive oil

Sea salt and freshly ground black pepper

1 head butter lettuce

1 head radicchio

1 large Honey Crisp, Gala, or Fuji apple, cored and thinly sliced

In a small bowl, mix the blue cheese, vinegar, and olive oil. Season to taste with salt and pepper.

In a large salad bowl, combine the lettuce and radicchio with the apple slices. Toss with the dressing and serve immediately. SERVES 6

citrus-marinated barbecued shrimp with fresh arugula

PROTEIN, HEALTHY FATS, VEGETABLES

DETOX, LEVEL 1, LEVEL 2

For the shrimp: Combine all the ingredients in a nonreactive bowl. Marinate the shrimp for 30 minutes. Prepare the grill. Cook the shrimp over a hot grill, basting with the marinade until just cooked through. Do not overcook the shrimp, or they will get tough. Keep warm.

   For the arugula: Toss the arugula with the olive oil, lemon juice, and salt and pepper. Arrange on four plates. To serve, position the shrimp in a lovely pattern on top of the arugula.   SERVES 4

SHRIMP

20 large shrimp, peeled and deveined

7 garlic cloves, pressed

1 bunch cilantro, chopped

1/2 cup olive oil

3 serrano chiles, chopped (see Note, page 39)

Zest from 1 lime

Juice from 3 limes

ARUGULA

1 pound fresh arugula, tough stems removed

2 teaspoons extra virgin olive oil

Juice from 1 lemon

Sea salt and freshly ground black pepper

spicy rock shrimp salad

PROTEIN, VEGETABLES

DETOX, LEVEL 1, LEVEL 2

1 pound peeled rock
shrimp (see Note)

Sea salt and white
pepper

¹/₂ cup Thai fish sauce
(nam pla)

1 cup fresh lime juice

¹/₂ cup white vinegar

¹/₂ cup clam juice

1 red onion, finely diced

3 serrano chiles, finely
minced, with seeds
(see Note, page 39)

2 ripe tomatoes, peeled,
seeded, and diced

2 pickling cucumbers,
diced with skins on

1 bunch cilantro

Dash of hot pepper
sauce

1 head green leaf
lettuce, leaves
separated

Sprinkle the shrimp with salt and white pepper. Blanch in boiling water for 2 to 3 minutes. Drain and chill.

Combine the fish sauce, lime juice, vinegar, clam juice, onion, chiles, tomatoes, cucumbers, and cilantro. Toss well with the chilled rock shrimp. Season with hot pepper sauce and salt and pepper.

Using a slotted spoon, place a chilled mound of the shrimp salad over the green leaf lettuce.   SERVES 6

NOTE Rock shrimp usually come raw and peeled. They cook very quickly. Simply place in salted boiling water until they turn pink. Remove immediately and drain.

salade niçoise

PROTEIN, HEALTHY FATS, VEGETABLES
DETOX, LEVEL 1, LEVEL 2

Season the tuna with salt and pepper. Heat the oil in a large sauté pan over medium-high heat. Add the garlic. Brown the garlic for 2 to 3 minutes, then add the tuna. Cook the tuna for 3 to 4 minutes on each side. Remove the tuna and garlic from the pan and keep them warm in a 200°F oven. Add the onion rings to the pan, stirring until they wilt.

Toss the beans and celery root in about 2 tablespoons of the vinaigrette. Arrange the dressed vegetables in the centers of two salad plates. Place the tuna and garlic on the vegetables. Drizzle with the vinaigrette, then mound the red onions on top of the tuna. Arrange the tomato wedges and hard-boiled eggs on the side. Sprinkle with chopped parsley and serve. SERVES 2

Two 4-ounce fresh ahi tuna fillets

Sea salt and freshly ground black pepper

1 tablespoon olive oil

2 garlic cloves, thickly sliced

1 small red onion, sliced in rings

8 ounces green beans, trimmed and steamed

1 small celery root, peeled, cubed, and steamed

1 cup Lemon Tarragon Vinaigrette (page 144)

1 Roma (plum) tomato, cut into 4 wedges

2 hard-boiled eggs, sliced in half

2 tablespoons finely chopped flat-leaf parsley

warm frisée salad with poached egg and pancetta

2 tablespoons extra
virgin olive oil

$1/4$ cup diced pancetta

1 head frisée or other
hearty lettuce, cut
into 1-inch pieces

$1/2$ tablespoon sherry
vinegar

Sea salt and freshly
ground black pepper

2 large eggs

PROTEIN, HEALTHY FATS, VEGETABLES

DETOX, LEVEL 1, LEVEL 2

In a large sauté pan over medium heat, place 1 tablespoon of the oil and the pancetta. Cook slowly until rendered and crispy. Add the frisée and toss with the remaining tablespoon of oil. Allow the frisée to wilt slightly. Add the vinegar, salt, and pepper. Remove from the heat and set aside.

In a small saucepan over high heat, boil 3 cups of water. Reduce the heat to a simmer and crack the eggs into the water. Cook for 3 to 4 minutes or until desired doneness.

Put the salad on two plates and place an egg atop each portion. Serve immediately.   SERVES 2

cobb salad

PROTEIN, HEALTHY FATS, VEGETABLES
DETOX, LEVEL 1, LEVEL 2

Place the lettuce in a large salad bowl and toss with the vinaigrette.

Arrange the tossed lettuce on four large salad plates. Top the greens with a vertical row of the zucchini, then a row of bacon, diced egg, diced tomato, cheese, turkey, and scallion slices. Or, for a tossed Cobb salad, toss all the ingredients in the salad bowl and serve. SERVES 4

1 pound mixed salad greens

$^3/_4$ cup Herb Vinaigrette (page 144)

1 small zucchini, diced

4 bacon strips, cooked until crisp and crumbled

2 large eggs, hard-boiled and diced

1 ripe medium tomato, diced

8 ounces crumbled blue cheese, preferably Maytag or Roquefort

$^1/_4$ pound smoked turkey breast, diced

2 scallions, white and green parts, thinly sliced

caesar salad

CAESAR DRESSING

4 anchovy fillets

1 teaspoon cracked black peppercorns

⅓ cup extra virgin olive oil

½ cup freshly grated Parmesan cheese

1 large egg, preferably pasteurized

3 tablespoons red wine vinegar

2 tablespoons fresh lemon juice

1 tablespoon pureed garlic

2 teaspoons dry mustard

1 teaspoon celery salt

3 dashes Tabasco sauce

3 dashes Worcestershire sauce (see Note, page 45)

2 medium heads romaine lettuce, or 4 hearts of romaine

Shavings of Parmesan cheese, for garnish

For the dressing: Combine the anchovies, black pepper, and olive oil in a mixing cup or blender jar. Using a hand mixer (or the blender), puree until very smooth, 1 to 2 minutes. Add the Parmesan and blend briefly to combine.

Bring a small saucepan of water to a boil. Place the egg on a slotted spoon and lower it into the boiling water. Cook for 1½ minutes, remove, and reserve.

Place the remaining dressing ingredients in a large bowl and whisk in the anchovy mixture. Crack open the egg and spoon the contents (including the parts that are uncooked) into the bowl. Whisk until well combined. (The dressing may be refrigerated at this stage.)

For the salad: Wash and dry the lettuce. Arrange the lettuce spears on serving plates and drizzle the dressing over the top. Garnish with shaved Parmesan, and serve. SERVES 6

parmesan bowls with caesar salad

PROTEIN, HEALTHY FATS, VEGETABLES
DETOX, LEVEL 1, LEVEL 2

1¹/₂ cups freshly grated
  Parmesan cheese
Caesar Salad (page 86)

For the Parmesan bowls: Set out four small soup bowls or four small "jelly jar" style glasses. Turn the soup bowls or glasses upside down on the counter.

Place an 8-inch nonstick skillet on medium heat.

Sprinkle one-fourth of the cheese into the skillet and quickly spread it around until it is evenly dispersed. When the cheese starts to bubble, about 3 minutes, gently lift with a nonstick spatula and turn over to brown on the other side, another 2 to 3 minutes. Slide the cheese "pancake" out of the pan and onto the upside-down soup bowl or glass. Gently press to conform to the shape of the soup bowl or glass. Let sit for a few minutes, while you make remaining pancakes.

When ready to serve, place the prepared salad into the Parmesan "bowls."

MAKES 4 BOWLS

NOTE For a mini Parmesan bowl, begin with a 4-inch Parmesan pancake and cool it over a shot glass. This will create an individual, appetizer-size bowl.

grilled chicken caesar salad

PROTEIN, HEALTHY FATS, VEGETABLES
DETOX, LEVEL 1, LEVEL 2

Six 6-ounce skinless
  and boneless
  chicken breasts
Sea salt and freshly
  ground black pepper
2 tablespoons extra
  virgin olive oil
Caesar Salad (page 86)
1 lemon, cut into
  6 wedges, for
  garnish

Season the chicken with salt and pepper. Cook over a hot grill, about 4 minutes per side, brushing with olive oil. (The chicken can be pan-fried if you don't have a grill.) Remove from the heat and set aside.

Prepare the Caesar Salad and toss with most of the dressing, reserving a few tablespoons dressing to drizzle over the chicken.

Arrange the salad on six plates. Slice the chicken on the diagonal into ¼-inch-thick slices. Fan on top of the salad. Drizzle the remaining dressing over the chicken. Garnish with a lemon wedge. Season with additional salt and pepper. SERVES 6

grilled chicken salad with watercress and blue cheese vinaigrette

PROTEIN, HEALTHY FATS, VEGETABLES

DETOX, LEVEL 1, LEVEL 2

Four 6-ounce skinless and boneless chicken breasts

Sea salt and freshly ground black pepper

2 tablespoons extra virgin olive oil

1 head red leaf lettuce, leaves rinsed and dried

2 bunches watercress, rinsed and dried

3/4 cup Blue Cheese Vinaigrette (page 145)

1 pint yellow cherry tomatoes, for garnish

Season the chicken with salt and pepper. Cook over a hot grill, about 4 minutes per side, brushing with olive oil. Remove from the heat and set aside.

Tear the lettuce and watercress into small pieces and toss with most of the vinaigrette, reserving a few tablespoons dressing to drizzle over the chicken.

Arrange the greens on four plates. Slice the chicken on the diagonal into ¼-inch-thick slices. Fan on top of the greens. Drizzle the remaining vinaigrette over the chicken. Garnish with halved cherry tomatoes. Season to taste with additional salt and pepper.   SERVES 4

grilled chicken salad with sun-dried tomatoes and goat cheese

PROTEIN, HEALTHY FATS, VEGETABLES

DETOX, LEVEL 1, LEVEL 2

Season the chicken with salt and pepper. Cook over a hot grill, about 4 minutes per side, brushing with olive oil. Remove from heat and set aside.

Tear the lettuce into small pieces and toss with the sun-dried tomatoes and vinaigrette, reserving a few tablespoons dressing to drizzle over the chicken and cheese.

Arrange the lettuce on four plates. Slice the chicken on the diagonal into ¼-inch-thick slices. Fan on top of the lettuce. Arrange 2 slices of goat cheese on each plate. Drizzle the remaining vinaigrette over the chicken and cheese. Season to taste with additional salt and pepper.   SERVES 4

Four 6-ounce skinless and boneless chicken breasts

Sea salt and freshly ground black pepper

2 tablespoons olive oil

2 heads butter lettuce, leaves rinsed and dried

½ cup sun-dried tomatoes, drained and chopped

½ cup Balsamic Vinaigrette (page 143)

10 ounces goat cheese, sliced into 8 rounds

achiote chicken with radish and cucumber salad

PROTEIN, HEALTHY FATS, VEGETABLES

DETOX, LEVEL 1, LEVEL 2

CHICKEN

2 tablespoons ground achiote

2 tablespoons olive oil

Juice from 1 lime

Sea salt and freshly ground black pepper

Two 6-ounce skinless and boneless chicken breasts

SALAD

1 bunch radishes, sliced into quarters

1 cucumber, peeled, seeded, and cut into half-moons

1 bunch arugula or spinach

Extra virgin olive oil

Sherry vinegar

Sea salt and freshly ground black pepper

For the chicken: Preheat the oven to 400°F.

In a mixing bowl, combine all the ingredients except the chicken. Mix until smooth. Place the chicken into a nonreactive bowl, add the marinade, and let sit for 15 minutes (or up to 24 hours in the refrigerator).

Remove the chicken from the marinade and place in a baking pan. Roast until thoroughly cooked, about 20 minutes. Remove from the oven and allow to cool completely. When cooled, slice on the diagonal.

For the salad: In a mixing bowl, combine the radishes, cucumber, and arugula. Drizzle lightly with olive oil and a splash of vinegar. Season to taste with salt and pepper and toss until well coated.

Place the salad greens on individual plates and top with sliced chicken. Serve immediately.   SERVES 2

chopped salami and vegetable salad

PROTEIN, HEALTHY FATS, VEGETABLES

DETOX, LEVEL 1, LEVEL 2

Combine the lettuce, salami, cheese, and vegetables in a large bowl. Toss with the dressing. Arrange the salad on four plates. Add 2 pepperoncini to each salad. Season to taste with salt and pepper.   SERVES 4

1 head iceberg lettuce, rinsed, dried, and chopped

¼ pound Italian dry salami, thinly sliced, then cut into thin strips

¼ pound mozzarella cheese, thinly sliced, then cut into thin strips

10 medium white mushrooms, thinly sliced, then cut into thin strips

1 red bell pepper, stemmed, seeded, and julienned

½ cup French Dressing (page 145)

8 whole pepperoncini, for garnish

Sea salt and freshly ground black pepper

taco salad

2 tablespoons olive oil

1 medium onion, chopped

5 garlic cloves, pressed

1 pound ground beef

1 teaspoon paprika

1 teaspoon ground cumin

1/2 teaspoon dried oregano

1/2 teaspoon chili powder

1/2 teaspoon cayenne

Sea salt and freshly ground black pepper

One 6-ounce can tomato paste

1 head romaine lettuce, leaves rinsed, dried, and chopped

2 ripe medium tomatoes, chopped

6 ounces Cheddar cheese, grated

6 tablespoons sour cream

6 scallions, white and green parts, sliced

One 8-ounce jar salsa

Heat the oil in a large skillet over medium heat. Add the onion and cook until translucent, about 4 minutes. Add the garlic and cook for 1 minute longer. Turn up the heat to high and add the ground beef. Brown the meat, stirring constantly, until crumbly, about 4 minutes. Drain excess fat. Lower heat and add the paprika, cumin, oregano, chili powder, cayenne, and plenty of salt and pepper. Add 1 cup water and the tomato paste, blending well with a wooden spoon. Bring to a boil, then reduce the heat to low and simmer for 10 minutes, stirring occasionally.

Place the chopped romaine on four plates. Spoon the meat mixture over the lettuce. Top with the tomatoes, cheese, sour cream, scallions, and a spoonful of salsa.   SERVES 4

chopped vegetable salad with roasted chicken

PROTEIN, HEALTHY FATS, VEGETABLES

DETOX, LEVEL 1, LEVEL 2

Preheat the oven to 450°F.

Season the chicken liberally with salt and pepper. Place a large ovenproof sauté pan over medium-high heat. Add the olive oil and chicken and sear for 3 minutes per side. Place the sauté pan in the oven and roast for 5 to 6 minutes. When done, brush the chicken with some vinaigrette. Remove the chicken from the pan and set aside to cool. When cool, dice the chicken into ½-inch chunks.

In a mixing bowl, toss the mixed greens with 2 tablespoons of the vinaigrette until well coated. Divide the greens among four salad plates.

Place all the chopped vegetables and chicken in the bowl. Season with salt and pepper. Add the remaining vinaigrette and toss until well coated. Place the chicken and vegetable mixture on top of the greens and serve immediately.   SERVES 4

Four 6-ounce skinless and boneless chicken breasts

Sea salt and freshly ground black pepper

2 tablespoons olive oil

1 cup Champagne Mustard Vinaigrette (page 142)

1 pound mixed baby greens

1 red bell pepper, seeded and medium diced

1 yellow bell pepper, seeded and medium diced

1 medium cucumber, peeled, seeded, and medium diced

2 celery stalks, medium diced

½ red onion, medium diced

2 scallions, white and green parts, sliced

southern country fried chicken salad

1 head romaine lettuce, washed and chopped

2 medium cucumbers, peeled and sliced

3 celery stalks, chopped

2 to 3 cups coconut oil

Four 6-ounce skinless and boneless chicken breasts, chopped into 1-inch cubes

Sea salt and freshly ground black pepper

3/4 cup Green Goddess Dressing (page 146)

1 pint cherry tomatoes

Handful of toasted pecans (omit for Detox)

Handful of corn kernels off the cob (omit for Detox and Level 1)

Place the lettuce in a large bowl. Add the cucumbers and celery.

Heat the oil in a deep skillet on medium-high heat. Season the chicken pieces with salt and pepper. Add the chicken to the hot oil and fry for about 5 minutes, until golden brown. Drain on paper towels.

Toss the lettuce with the dressing. Top with the chicken pieces and garnish with cherry tomatoes, and the pecans and corn kernels, if using. Serve immediately.   SERVES 2

chinese chicken salad

For the dressing: Place the rice vinegar, lemon juice, soy sauce, and pepper to taste in a mixing cup. Add the olive oil and sesame oil in a steady stream, whisking constantly until the oil is emulsified. Set aside.

For the marinated chicken: Slice the chicken into bite-size pieces. Place in a nonreactive bowl with the remaining marinade ingredients and marinate 2 to 24 hours. The longer you marinate, the more intense the flavors.

To finish: Heat a wok over high heat. Add the coconut oil and chicken pieces. Sauté the chicken for about 3 minutes, until cooked through. Set aside.

Toss the greens with the dressing. Arrange on four plates, then place the hot chicken pieces on the greens. Add the beans, season with freshly ground pepper, and serve.   SERVES 4

DRESSING

2 tablespoons rice vinegar

Juice of $1/2$ lemon

1 tablespoon soy sauce

Freshly ground black pepper

5 tablespoons extra virgin olive oil

1 tablespoon toasted sesame oil

MARINATED CHICKEN

Four 6-ounce boneless and skinless chicken breasts

$1/4$ cup soy sauce

$1/4$ cup toasted sesame oil

$1/2$ teaspoon hot chili oil

3 garlic cloves, pressed

1 tablespoon grated fresh ginger, or 1 teaspoon dried

Juice of 1 lemon

TO FINISH

1 tablespoon coconut oil

1 pound mixed field greens

1 recipe Chinese Long Beans (page 163)

Freshly ground black pepper

pork medallions over pale greens with pepper-thyme vinaigrette

PROTEIN, HEALTHY FATS, VEGETABLES
DETOX, LEVEL 1, LEVEL 2

PORK MEDALLIONS

2 pork tenderloins

1/2 cup olive oil

Juice from 1 lemon

2 teaspoons fresh
   thyme leaves

PEPPER-THYME
VINAIGRETTE

Juice from 2 lemons

1 teaspoon sea salt

1/2 cup extra virgin
   olive oil

1/4 cup black
   peppercorns

6 shallots, very finely
   chopped

1 teaspoon fresh
   thyme leaves

TO FINISH

1 head Bibb lettuce,
   leaves separated,
   washed, and dried

2 heads frisée (baby
   curly endive),
   washed and dried

1 1/2 cups cherry
   tomatoes

For the pork: Rinse and pat dry the tenderloins. Slice on the diagonal into ¼-inch medallions. Place them in a nonreactive container and marinate in the olive oil, lemon juice, and thyme for 2 hours, refrigerated, turning after 1 hour.

For the vinaigrette: Place the lemon juice in a small bowl. Add the salt, then the olive oil in a thin, steady stream, whisking constantly. On a chopping block, crack the peppercorns using a frying pan. Combine the cracked peppercorns, shallots, and thyme with two-thirds of the lemon-oil mixture. Set remaining one-third aside.

In a hot frying pan over medium-high heat, cook the pork approximately 2 minutes per side (do not overcook, or it will get dry and tough). The pork should be just cooked through, juicy with a hint of pink in the center.

To finish: Toss the greens with the reserved lemon-oil mixture. Arrange on four plates. Fan the pork medallions over the greens and top with a generous amount of the vinaigrette. Garnish with cherry tomatoes and serve immediately.   SERVES 4

warm steak and arugula salad
with parmesan shavings

PROTEIN, HEALTHY FATS, VEGETABLES

DETOX, LEVEL 1, LEVEL 2

4 tablespoons extra
   virgin olive oil

1 tablespoon balsamic
   vinegar

Sea salt and freshly
   ground black pepper

4 ounces arugula

1 pint cherry tomatoes,
   cut in half

1 pound beef tip steak

Shavings of Parmesan
   cheese

Whisk 3 tablespoons of the olive oil in a bowl with the balsamic vinegar. Season with salt and pepper. Add the arugula and tomatoes, and toss to coat. Place on a large serving platter or four dinner plates.

Pat the steak dry with paper towels. Season liberally with salt and pepper. Heat a large sauté pan on medium-high heat. Add the remaining tablespoon olive oil, then the steak. Sauté the steak until browned, about 5 minutes on each side.

Place steak on a cutting board. Allow to rest for 3 minutes, then thinly slice against the grain. Arrange the hot steak slices over the arugula. Top with Parmesan shavings before serving.   SERVES 4

thai beef with cucumber salad

CUCUMBER SALAD

1 medium cucumber, peeled

1 tablespoon grated fresh ginger

1 tablespoon finely chopped fresh mint

1/2 red onion, thinly sliced

1/4 cup rice wine vinegar

1 teaspoon All Natural SomerSweet

Sea salt and freshly ground black pepper

THAI BEEF

2 tablespoons olive oil

1 Thai chile (or serrano or jalapeño), thinly sliced (see Note, page 39)

1/2 bunch fresh mint leaves, chopped

1 tablespoon finely chopped cilantro

4 fresh basil leaves, julienned

Juice and zest of 1/4 lime

One 8-ounce filet mignon or rib-eye steak

For the cucumber salad: Slice the cucumber in half lengthwise, scrape out the seeds, then cut into half-moon pieces. Toss in a bowl with the ginger, mint, onion, vinegar, and All Natural SomerSweet. Season with salt and pepper. Set aside to let the flavors combine.

For the Thai beef: Combine 1 tablespoon of the olive oil, the chile, mint, cilantro, basil, lime juice, and lime zest in a large nonreactive bowl. Add the beef and marinate for 30 minutes.

In a medium sauté pan, heat the remaining 1 tablespoon of olive oil over high heat, then sear the beef for 2 minutes on each side for medium-rare. Remove from the heat and let rest for 2 minutes. Thinly slice against the grain.

Place steak slices on individual plates. Top each with a mound of cucumber salad. SERVES 2

turkey salad in lettuce cups

PROTEIN, HEALTHY FATS, VEGETABLES

DETOX, LEVEL 1, LEVEL 2

Place the turkey, mayonnaise, celery, scallions (reserve a few scallions for garnish), and salt and pepper in a bowl and mix until well combined. Adjust the seasonings to taste.

Place a large dollop of turkey salad in each lettuce leaf, then garnish with the reserved scallions. Add a spoonful of cranberry sauce as an additional garnish, if using. Fold up and eat like a taco.

MAKES 4 TO 6 LETTUCE CUPS

2 cups chopped cooked turkey

3 tablespoons mayonnaise

3 celery stalks, finely chopped

5 scallions, white and green parts, finely chopped

Sea salt and freshly ground black pepper

4 to 6 iceberg lettuce leaves

Cranberry sauce (for Level 2 only)

tuna salad in lettuce cups

PROTEIN, HEALTHY FATS, VEGETABLES

DETOX, LEVEL 1, LEVEL 2

Place the tuna, mayonnaise, celery, red onion, lemon juice, pepper, and dill in a bowl and mix until well combined. Adjust the seasonings.

Place a large dollop of tuna salad in each lettuce leaf, then garnish with tomatoes and scallions. Fold up and eat like a taco.

MAKES 4 TO 6 CUPS

One 12-ounce can tuna, drained white albacore packed in water

4 tablespoons mayonnaise

3 celery stalks, finely chopped

1/2 red onion, finely chopped

Juice from 1 lemon

Freshly ground black pepper

1/2 teaspoon dried dill

4 to 6 iceberg lettuce leaves

2 or 3 plum tomatoes, chopped

3 scallions, white and green parts, sliced

tarragon chicken salad in lettuce cups

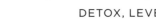

PROTEIN, HEALTHY FATS, VEGETABLES

DETOX, LEVEL 1, LEVEL 2

2 cups chopped cooked chicken

3 tablespoons mayonnaise

3 celery stalks, finely chopped

1/4 sweet onion (Vidalia or Maui), finely chopped

2 tablespoons chopped fresh tarragon, or 1/2 teaspoon dried

Sea salt and freshly ground black pepper

4 to 6 romaine lettuce leaves

3 scallions, white and green parts, sliced

Sprigs of fresh tarragon, for garnish

Place chicken, mayonnaise, celery, onion, chopped tarragon, and salt and pepper in a bowl and mix until well combined. Adjust seasonings to taste.

Place a large dollop of chicken salad in each lettuce leaf, then garnish with the scallions and tarragon sprigs. Fold up and eat like a taco.

MAKES 4 TO 6 CUPS

egg salad in lettuce cups

PROTEIN, HEALTHY FATS, VEGETABLES

DETOX, LEVEL 1, LEVEL 2

Place the eggs in a saucepan filled with enough cold water to cover them. Bring the water to a boil, then lower the heat to medium and cook for 15 minutes. Drain the hot water and run the hard-boiled eggs under cold water until cool enough to peel.

Dice the peeled eggs and place in a large bowl. Add the mayonnaise, celery, chopped chives, and salt and pepper. Combine well, adjusting the seasonings.

Place a large dollop of egg salad in each lettuce leaf, then garnish with a few onion sprouts, if desired, and chives. Fold up and eat like a taco. MAKES 4 TO 6 CUPS

8 large eggs

4 tablespoons mayonnaise

3 celery stalks, finely chopped

10 chives or 5 scallions, white parts only, finely chopped

Sea salt and freshly ground black pepper

4 to 6 butter lettuce leaves

Handful of onion sprouts (optional)

Chives, for garnish

radicchio cups with curried chicken

2 tablespoons Thai red curry paste

1 teaspoon yellow curry powder

3 tablespoons extra virgin olive oil

1 lime

3 chicken thighs, boned

1 cup chicken stock or broth, preferably homemade (pages 30–32)

¼ cup mayonnaise

Sea salt and freshly ground black pepper

3 heads radicchio, leaves washed and separated

Chives, for garnish

In a glass or other nonreactive bowl, mix the curry paste and curry powder with 2 tablespoons of the olive oil and the juice from ½ of the lime. Place the chicken in the marinade and refrigerate for 30 minutes, turning once to evenly coat.

Preheat the oven to 375°F.

Place an ovenproof sauté pan over medium heat and add the remaining 1 tablespoon of olive oil. Sear the chicken for 3 minutes on each side. Add the stock and bring to a boil. Cover the pan with a lid and place in the oven to roast until the chicken is cooked through, about 30 minutes. Remove the chicken from the pan and allow to cool, reserving the juices. When cool enough to handle, chop the chicken into small pieces and reserve 1 tablespoon of the liquid.

In a small bowl, mix the mayonnaise and reserved liquid. Add the chicken and season to taste with salt, pepper, and a squeeze of juice from the remaining ½ lime.

Use each radicchio leaf as a cup. Trim with kitchen scissors, if necessary. Spoon the chicken filling into the radicchio cups, garnish with a crisscross of chives, and serve immediately. MAKES 16 CUPS

appetizers, sandwiches, and sides

something special

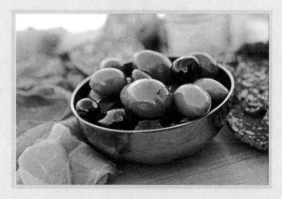

An appetizer . . . it's a taste. Something special and small. While perusing menus at restaurants, I am usually most enticed by the appetizers. I find myself ordering two or three instead of an entrée. At parties, I love the cocktail hour most, mingling and sharing fabulous little nibbles passed on trays or set out in visually appealing designs. The appetizer, the starter to whet the appetite; it prepares the palate for what's to come. An appetizer can also be a seated first course. Either way, it's the introduction to the meal.

I don't discriminate from fancy to casual. Sure, I love caviar, but a plate of Buffalo Wings with Blue Cheese Dip (page 115) also holds a special place in my heart. A beautiful cheese plate might be my absolute favorite. Make sure to try the Parmesan Crisps (page 107), my ingenious alternative to a cracker. The Grilled Scallops Wrapped in Prosciutto with Basil-Parsley Pesto (page 125) will rock your world. Mini Burgers with Gorgonzola and Caramelized Onions (page 117) are always a crowd favorite. Some of these recipes are labor intensive, like the Mini Lettuce Cups with Minced Duck (page 113), but they are worth it. I will never forget Tom Ford's face when he bit into one. He designs clothes. I design flavor. Reciprocity.

I've also included a few favorite sandwiches and several special sides. I highly recommend you try the Candied Tomato Tart (page 135), based on the years I spent in Provence. Have the family or your guests sitting at the table when you make my famous (at least in my family!) Whole Wheat Popovers (page 135). They come out of the oven all puffed and fluffy and *amazing*! Serve with a salad and you will have a memorable meal. For those on my Sexy Forever Weight Loss Plan, reserve these for Level 2, and enjoy the rewards of reaching your goal weight. You deserve to love life and enjoy indulgences while keeping your slim waist.

crostini with homemade ricotta cheese

HEALTHY FATS, CARBOHYDRATES

LEVEL 1, LEVEL 2

Place the cream, milk, and yogurt in a medium saucepan and heat over medium heat. Stir frequently until small bubbles form around the edge. Lower the heat and simmer for 20 minutes. Turn off the heat and allow to cool so that the whey (the watery liquid) and curds separate. Line a strainer with cheesecloth and ladle the ricotta into it. Allow the liquid to drain out of the cheese curds for a few minutes; then draw up the sides of the cheesecloth and scrape the ricotta into a bowl. Season with a little salt.

Toast the bread until golden brown. Spread the ricotta on the toast and serve. (Place any remaining ricotta in an airtight container and store in the refrigerator for up to 1 week.) SERVES 2

1 cup heavy cream

1 cup whole milk

$\frac{1}{4}$ cup full-fat, plain yogurt

Sea salt

2 thin slices hard-crusted whole-grain bread

whole-grain crostini with goat cheese and candied tomato relish

HEALTHY FATS, VEGETABLES, CARBOHYDRATES

LEVEL 1, LEVEL 2

Chop the tomatoes into small pieces. Mix in a bowl with the basil and olive oil and season with salt and pepper.

Thinly slice the bread to create 2 × 4-inch pieces. Brush the bread with olive oil and toast in the oven or a toaster oven until lightly browned. Smear with the goat cheese and top with the tomato relish. MAKES 16

6 Candied Tomatoes (page 174)

2 tablespoons julienned basil leaves

2 tablespoons extra virgin olive oil, plus more for brushing

Sea salt and freshly ground black pepper

1 loaf crusty whole-grain bread

6 ounces fresh goat cheese

mozzarella marinara

PROTEIN, HEALTHY FATS, VEGETABLES

DETOX, LEVEL 1, LEVEL 2

1 pound mozzarella cheese

2 large eggs, lightly beaten

¾ cup freshly grated Parmesan cheese

1 recipe Sweet Tomato Sauce (page 183) or your favorite marinara

Slice the cheese across the width into slices ½ inch thick. Dip each slice of cheese in the beaten egg, then coat in Parmesan cheese. Place the prepared cheese slices on a plate and freeze them until just before you are ready to cook them.

Preheat the broiler.

Warm the tomato sauce in a small saucepan.

Arrange the frozen cheese slices on a baking sheet. Place the baking sheet under the broiler for 2 to 3 minutes, until the cheese starts to bubble and turn golden brown. Carefully flip over each cheese slice with a spatula and brown the other side.

Place each slice on a plate and top with warm tomato sauce. Serve immediately. SERVES 4 TO 6

parmesan crisps with prosciutto and arugula

PROTEIN, HEALTHY FATS, VEGETABLES

DETOX, LEVEL 1, LEVEL 2

8 thin slices prosciutto, cut in half across

Handful of baby arugula

Truffle oil or extra virgin olive oil

16 Parmesan Crisps (recipe follows)

Freshly ground black pepper

Place a piece of prosciutto, a leaf of arugula, and a drizzle of truffle oil on each Parmesan crisp. Season with pepper. SERVES 4

parmesan crisps

HEALTHY FATS

DETOX, LEVEL 1, LEVEL 2

1/2 cup finely shredded
Parmesan cheese

Preheat the oven to 350°F.

Line a baking sheet with parchment paper (or use a Silpat nonstick mat). Sprinkle the cheese into 3-inch circles, making several mini "pancakes." Place in the oven and bake for about 5 minutes, until just golden. Remove from the oven and let cool slightly. MAKES 16 CRISPS

melted burrata cheese with roasted eggplant and basil in parmesan bowls

HEALTHY FATS, VEGETABLES

DETOX, LEVEL 1, LEVEL 2

3 Japanese eggplants

Extra virgin olive oil

Sea salt and freshly
ground black pepper

1 cup fresh shredded
Burrata cheese or
mozzarella

1/2 cup tomato sauce,
warmed

16 mini Parmesan bowls
(see page 87)

2 tablespoons julienned
basil, for garnish

Preheat the oven to 350°F.

Trim and quarter the eggplants lengthwise into spears. Drizzle with olive oil, season with salt and pepper, and place on a baking sheet. Roast until soft, 20 to 25 minutes. Remove from the oven. When cool enough to handle, cut into medium dice.

On another baking sheet, create 16 small piles of eggplant, about 2 pieces of eggplant per pile. Top each with about ½ tablespoon of the cheese. Bake for about 5 minutes, or until the cheese melts.

To assemble, place a dollop of tomato sauce into each Parmesan bowl, then use a spatula to scrape the eggplant and cheese into the bowl. Garnish with the basil and serve immediately. MAKES 16 BOWLS

whole wheat crostini with red pepper rouille

Extra virgin olive oil, for drizzling

4 slices crusty, whole wheat bread

¾ cup Red Pepper Rouille (page 152)

HEALTHY FATS, VEGETABLES, CARBOHYDRATES

LEVEL 1, LEVEL 2

Drizzle olive oil onto the bread slices and broil or grill until golden. Cut each slice on the diagonal and drizzle the toast with the rouille.

MAKES 8 CROSTINI

endive spears with apple, prosciutto, and gorgonzola

Olive oil

4 slices prosciutto, julienned

16 Belgian endive spears, washed

1 cup baby spinach leaves, julienned

1 head radicchio, julienned

1 Fuji or Gala apple, julienned (omit for Detox and Level 1)

4 ounces Gorgonzola cheese, cut into small pieces

Sea salt and freshly ground black pepper

PROTEIN, HEALTHY FATS, VEGETABLES, FRUIT

DETOX, LEVEL 1, LEVEL 2

In a medium sauté pan, add olive oil to cover the bottom of the pan and heat on medium high. Add the prosciutto and cook until crisp. Remove from the oil and drain on paper towels.

To assemble, lay endive spears on a platter and top each spear with small amounts of spinach, radicchio, apple, if using, prosciutto, and a sprinkling of cheese. Season with salt and pepper. Serve immediately. MAKES 16 SPEARS

stuffed mushrooms

HEALTHY FATS, VEGETABLES

DETOX, LEVEL 1, LEVEL 2

1 pound large white mushrooms

4 tablespoons ($\frac{1}{2}$ stick) unsalted butter

4 shallots, finely chopped

1 tablespoon chopped lemon thyme (or parsley or tarragon)

Sea salt and freshly ground black pepper

$\frac{1}{4}$ to $\frac{1}{2}$ cup dry white wine (use vegetable or chicken stock for Detox)

$\frac{1}{2}$ cup freshly grated Parmesan cheese

2 tablespoons olive oil

Trim the very ends off the mushroom stems and discard. Then carefully pull the stems off the mushrooms. The mushroom stems will be used as part of the stuffing. Finely chop the mushroom stems. Select the 12 largest mushroom caps and set aside. Thinly slice the remaining mushrooms, then chop.

Melt the butter in a large skillet over medium heat. Add the shallots and sauté until golden, about 5 minutes. Add the mushroom stems, chopped mushrooms, lemon thyme, and salt and pepper to taste. Sauté until the mushrooms are browned and crusty, about 10 minutes. Add the white wine and let it cook off for about 3 minutes, scraping the bits from the bottom of the pan to release the flavor. Remove from the heat.

Preheat the broiler.

Place the mushroom mixture in a mixing bowl with ¼ cup of the Parmesan cheese. Stir until well combined.

Lightly rub the reserved mushroom caps with olive oil and place on a cookie sheet with the cavity side up. Fill each cavity with a heaping mound of the mushroom stuffing. Sprinkle the remaining ¼ cup Parmesan over the top.

Place the cookie sheet under the broiler for approximately 5 minutes.

Keep a close eye on them. Cook until the cheese bubbles and the mushroom caps get a little brown. If your broiler is very hot, the cheese may start to burn before the mushroom caps are cooked. In that case, lower the rack to allow the mushrooms to cook longer without burning the tops. Transfer to a platter and serve sizzling hot. MAKES 12 CAPS

roasted mushrooms with spinach, cheese, and pancetta

PROTEIN, HEALTHY FATS, VEGETABLES

DETOX, LEVEL 1, LEVEL 2

16 whole mushroom caps, stems removed and discarded

Sea salt and freshly ground black pepper

2 tablespoons ($^1\!/_4$ stick) unsalted butter, cut into small pieces

1 tablespoon olive oil

1 pound fresh spinach, washed and stemmed

$^1\!/_2$ cup finely diced onion

$^1\!/_2$ cup finely diced pancetta or bacon

1 cup fresh goat cheese

Preheat the oven to 350°F.

Place the mushrooms, stem side up, in a baking dish. Season with salt and pepper and place a small piece of butter in the center of each cap. Bake until cooked through, about 20 minutes.

While the mushrooms are roasting, in a sauté pan over medium heat, add ½ tablespoon of the olive oil and the spinach. Sauté until the spinach is wilted. Set aside.

In another sauté pan over medium heat, use the remaining ½ table-spoon of oil to cook the onion and pancetta until the pancetta is rendered of fat and the onion is slightly caramelized. Drain excess fat and set aside.

When the mushrooms are cooked, remove them from the oven. When cool enough to handle, fill each with a spoonful of goat cheese, then top with spinach and the pancetta mixture. Serve immediately. MAKES 16 CAPS

wild mushroom risotto in mushroom caps

PROTEIN, HEALTHY FATS, VEGETABLES, INSULIN TRIGGERS

LEVEL 2

Preheat the oven to 375°F.

In an ovenproof dish, place the mushroom caps with the chicken stock and distribute 1 tablespoon butter over the mushrooms. Cover and bake for 25 minutes.

In a saucepan, bring the mushroom stock to a boil and reduce to a simmer to keep warm. Place a medium saucepan over medium-high heat. Add 2 tablespoons of the olive oil and the onion. Continuously stir the onion so it does not burn or caramelize. When the onion is soft, after about 5 minutes, add the sliced wild mushrooms and the remaining tablespoon of oil. Season with salt and pepper. Sauté for 10 to 15 minutes, until the mushrooms are browned and slightly crusty. Add the rice and stir to coat with oil, onion, and mushrooms. Add the wine and reduce until almost dry. Once the wine is reduced, add half of the stock while stirring constantly. As the liquid is absorbed, continue to slowly add the remainder while still stirring. Continue until the risotto is cooked through. Turn off the heat and add the remaining 2 tablespoons of butter and the Parmesan cheese. Stir gently to combine.

Remove the mushrooms from the oven and fill each cap with a spoonful of warm risotto. Garnish with the chervil. Serve immediately. MAKES 16 CAPS

16 whole mushroom caps, stems removed and discarded

1/4 cup chicken stock or broth, preferably homemade (pages 30–32)

3 tablespoons unsalted butter

3 cups mushroom stock or chicken stock or broth

3 tablespoons olive oil

1/2 yellow onion, finely diced

2 cups mixed wild mushrooms, thinly sliced (or regular mushrooms)

Sea salt and freshly ground black pepper

1 cup Arborio rice

1/2 cup dry white wine

1/2 cup finely grated Parmesan cheese

Fresh chervil leaves, for garnish

summer salad on a skewer

1 red onion, thinly sliced

¼ cup Champagne vinegar

1 teaspoon All Natural SomerSweet

Sea salt and freshly ground black pepper

¼ cup fresh raspberries

2 cups cubed (¾-inch) watermelon

1 bunch watercress, cleaned and picked over

1 tablespoon extra virgin olive oil

16 wooden skewers

Place the sliced onion into a bowl and add the vinegar, All Natural SomerSweet, salt, and pepper. Set aside for at least 15 minutes to pickle the onion.

Pass the raspberries through a fine sieve into a mixing bowl. Discard the seeds and pulp. Add the watermelon to the raspberries and season with salt and pepper. Add the pickled onion and toss gently to combine.

To assemble, place 1 large watercress leaf onto a skewer followed by a watermelon chunk. Continue until all skewers are complete. Arrange on a platter and sprinkle with the remaining pickled onion. Drizzle with the olive oil and serve immediately.   MAKES 16 SKEWERS

mini lettuce cups with minced duck

PROTEIN, HEALTHY FATS, VEGETABLES, CARBOHYDRATES

DETOX, LEVEL 1, LEVEL 2

Preheat the oven to 375°F.

Season the duck liberally with salt and pepper, then coat the duck in 1 tablespoon of the oil. Place the duck into a roasting pan, skin side down. Place into the oven and roast for 30 minutes, then turn the duck and roast for another 30 minutes. When fully cooked, remove from the pan and set aside to cool.

Prepare 16 lettuce cups by cutting leaves into 3- to 4-inch round disks using kitchen scissors. Set aside.

In a sauté pan over medium heat, add the remaining tablespoon of the olive oil and the garlic. Toast the garlic until lightly browned. Set aside.

Mince the duck, including the skin, into small pieces and place into a bowl. Add the toasted garlic and the remaining ingredients and toss until combined. Adjust the seasoning. Spoon into lettuce rounds and serve immediately. MAKES 16 CUPS

4 duck legs

Sea salt and freshly ground black pepper

2 tablespoons olive oil

1 head iceberg lettuce, washed

1 garlic clove, minced

2 scallions, white and some green parts, sliced

1 tablespoon soy sauce

1 teaspoon sesame oil

1/4 teaspoon Asian chili paste

Juice from 1/2 lime

2 tablespoons toasted pine nuts (omit for Detox)

chicken drummettes

2 pounds chicken wing
drummettes

$^1/_3$ cup olive oil

Juice from 3 lemons

10 garlic cloves, pressed

10 sprigs fresh thyme
leaves

1 bunch flat-leaf parsley,
chopped

1 tablespoon dried
rosemary leaves

$^1/_2$ teaspoon or more
cayenne

1 teaspoon paprika

Sea salt and freshly
ground black pepper

PROTEIN, HEALTHY FATS, VEGETABLES

DETOX, LEVEL 1, LEVEL 2

Combine all the ingredients in a glass or other nonreactive bowl. Let marinate for 1 hour or more.

Heat a grill until very hot. Place the drummettes on the grill and cook for about 10 minutes, turning constantly.

MAKES ABOUT 30 DRUMMETTES

buffalo wings with blue cheese dip

PROTEIN, HEALTHY FATS, VEGETABLES
DETOX, LEVEL 1, LEVEL 2

Place the drummettes in a bowl and toss with the salt, paprika, and cayenne.

Place the oil in a large skillet; it should measure about 2 inches in the bottom of the pan. Heat over medium heat until the oil reaches approximately 375°F.

Fry about 8 wings at a time in the hot oil until crisp, about 10 minutes. (If you have a deep fryer, you can fry more wings at the same time.) Remove from oil and drain on paper towels.

Heat the hot sauce and butter over medium-low heat until well combined.

Serve the wings with the hot sauce and blue cheese dip on the side, accompanied by the celery and zucchini sticks and broccoli florets.   MAKES 36 DRUMMETTES

NOTE Traditional buffalo wings are completely coated in the hot sauce, but to keep the wings crisp, serve them with the hot sauce on the side. Guests can control the amount of hot sauce on each bite. (Plus, your fingers don't get so messy.)

36 chicken wing drummettes

2 tablespoons sea salt

2 tablespoons paprika

1 tablespoon cayenne

3 cups coconut or grapeseed oil

$\frac{1}{3}$ cup hot pepper sauce, such as Cholula

2 tablespoons ($\frac{1}{4}$ stick) unsalted butter

$1\frac{1}{2}$ cups Blue Cheese Dip (page 146)

1 head celery, trimmed and cut into 5-inch sticks

1 medium zucchini, cut into 5-inch sticks

1 bunch broccoli, florets lightly steamed

curry chicken skewers

PROTEIN, HEALTHY FATS, VEGETABLES

LEVEL 1, LEVEL 2

3 tablespoons red curry paste

¹/₂ cup coconut milk

Juice from 1 lime

1 tablespoon olive oil

Sea salt and freshly ground black pepper

Two 6-ounce skinless and boneless chicken breasts, cut lengthwise into 4 pieces

1 recipe Roasted Eggplant Relish (recipe follows)

In a medium bowl, mix the curry paste, coconut milk, lime juice, and olive oil. Season with salt and pepper. Add the chicken and coat well. Cover and refrigerate for at least 1 hour or overnight.

Heat the grill.

Remove the chicken from the marinade and skewer with either presoaked wooden skewers or metal skewers. On the hot grill, cook until done, about 3 minutes on each side. Serve immediately with the eggplant relish. SERVES 2

roasted eggplant relish

HEALTHY FATS, VEGETABLES

DETOX, LEVEL 1, LEVEL 2

4 Japanese eggplants, cut in half lengthwise

1 tablespoon extra virgin olive oil, plus more for drizzling

Sea salt and freshly ground black pepper

¹/₂ teaspoon ground cumin

1 teaspoon chopped fresh mint

Juice from ¹/₄ lemon

Preheat the oven to 350°F.

Place the eggplants on a baking sheet and sprinkle with the olive oil, salt, and pepper. Bake until soft and cooked through, about 30 minutes. Remove from the oven and allow to cool. Dice the eggplants into 1-inch pieces. Mix in a bowl with the cumin, a drizzle of olive oil, the mint, and lemon juice. Serve immediately. MAKES 1 CUP

mini burgers with gorgonzola and caramelized onions

PROTEIN, HEALTHY FATS, VEGETABLES

DETOX, LEVEL 1, LEVEL 2

In a mixing bowl, combine the beef, onion, egg, salt, and pepper. Form into 1-inch balls, then flatten slightly to form patties and set aside.

In a sauté pan over medium-high heat, add the olive oil and sear the burgers until they are crispy and brown, about 2 minutes per side. Remove from the heat and transfer to a baking sheet.

Preheat the broiler. Top the burgers with Gorgonzola and place under the broiler to melt the cheese. Top with caramelized onions and serve immediately. MAKES 16 BURGERS

1 pound ground beef

¼ cup finely minced onion (preferably Vidalia or Maui)

1 large egg

Sea salt and freshly ground black pepper

1 tablespoon olive oil

6 ounces Gorgonzola, cut into 12 thin slices

Caramelized Onions (recipe follows)

caramelized onions

HEALTHY FATS, VEGETABLES

DETOX, LEVEL 1, LEVEL 2

Olive oil

2 large onions, preferably Maui, very thinly sliced

In a medium sauté pan over medium-high heat, add enough olive oil to coat the pan. Add the onion slices in one layer and cook until they become brown and golden, 7 to 10 minutes. Once they begin to caramelize on the bottom, stir and turn to caramelize the tops. Lower the heat and continue to cook until soft and caramelized throughout, another 10 to 20 minutes. SERVES 4

pesto fondue with sausages

PROTEIN, HEALTHY FATS, VEGETABLES

DETOX, LEVEL 1, LEVEL 2

1 recipe Basil-Parsley Pesto (page 150)

¼ cup extra virgin olive oil

4 to 6 Italian chicken sausages

In a fondue pot, begin to heat the pesto and olive oil.

In a skillet, fry the sausages until cooked through. Let cool slightly, then cut them into bite-size pieces.

When pesto is bubbling, skewer the sausage pieces and dip into the pesto.   SERVES 4

seared beef with lime-chile-mint dipping sauce

PROTEIN, HEALTHY FATS, VEGETABLES

DETOX, LEVEL 1, LEVEL 2

½ cup extra virgin olive oil

One ½-pound piece beef tenderloin (or favorite cut)

Sea salt and freshly ground black pepper

1 cup fresh mint leaves

1 serrano chile, chopped (see Note, page 39)

Juice from 1 lime

2 tablespoons light soy sauce

16 wooden skewers, soaked in water

Preheat the oven to 400°F.

In a medium sauté pan over high heat, add 1 tablespoon of the olive oil. Season the beef with salt and pepper and sear all over until nicely browned, about 4 minutes. Remove from the heat and set aside.

Combine the mint leaves and serrano chile in a mixing cup or blender jar. Using a hand mixer (or blender), slowly add the remaining olive oil and puree to make a smooth paste. Add the lime juice, season with salt and pepper, and mix well.

Cut the beef on the diagonal into ¼-inch slices. Thread each slice onto a skewer. When ready to serve, place the skewers into an oven-proof pan and drizzle with the soy sauce. Heat in the oven for 3 to 4 minutes. Serve immediately with the dipping sauce.   MAKES 16

lamb skewers with harissa dipping sauce

PROTEIN, HEALTHY FATS, VEGETABLES

DETOX, LEVEL 1, LEVEL 2

For the skewers: Cut the lamb into 1- to 2-inch bite-size strips. Toss with the remaining ingredients and marinate for 3 to 4 hours or overnight.

Preheat the grill to high heat.

For the harissa sauce: Combine all the ingredients in a blender or food processor and blend until smooth. (Makes 1½ cups.)

Place the lamb on skewers (1 piece per skewer), then grill or broil for 2 to 3 minutes, turning frequently. Serve with the harissa sauce.   MAKES 25 TO 30 SKEWERS

LAMB SKEWERS

3 pounds boneless lamb loin

2 tablespoons ground cumin

2 tablespoons ground coriander

2 teaspoons sea salt

⅓ cup olive oil

3 tablespoons minced garlic

25 to 30 wooden skewers, soaked in water

HARISSA SAUCE

2 Roasted Red Peppers (page 134), peeled

1 tablespoon ground cumin

1 teaspoon sweet paprika

2 teaspoons sea salt

2 tablespoons extra virgin olive oil

1 teaspoon fresh lemon juice

curried lamb skewers with mint-cilantro pesto

PROTEIN, HEALTHY FATS, VEGETABLES

DETOX, LEVEL 1, LEVEL 2

2 tablespoons Thai red
   curry paste

Sea salt and freshly
   ground black pepper

¼ cup olive oil

Juice from 1 lime

2 teaspoons yellow
   curry powder

1 pound boneless lamb
   loin, cut into 1-inch
   cubes

1 cup Mint-Cilantro
   Pesto (page 151)

16 wooden skewers,
   soaked in water

In a small bowl, whisk together the curry paste, salt, pepper, oil, lime juice, and curry powder. Transfer to a glass or other nonreactive bowl and add the lamb. Marinate in the refrigerator for 20 to 30 minutes, turning once to evenly coat.

Preheat a grill to medium.

Remove the lamb from the marinade and place onto the skewers. Grill until medium-rare, 3 to 4 minutes per side. Remove from the heat and serve with the chile paste. MAKES 16 SKEWERS

curried lamb with cucumber-mint sour cream in radicchio cups

PROTEIN, HEALTHY FATS, VEGETABLES

DETOX, LEVEL 1, LEVEL 2

For the lamb: Heat a large sauté pan over medium heat. Add the olive oil and onion, and cook until the onion is golden brown, about 5 minutes. Add the garlic and cook for 1 minute more. Add the lamb, and season the meat with the curry powder, cinnamon, salt, and pepper. Sauté over medium-high heat until the lamb is cooked through, about 15 minutes.

For the sour cream: Place all the ingredients into a bowl and mix them until well combined.

For the cups: Fill each radicchio leaf with a large spoonful of curried lamb. Top with sour cream sauce and garnish with a mint leaf. Fold up and eat like a taco.   SERVES 8

CURRIED LAMB
2 tablespoons olive oil

1 medium onion, chopped

2 garlic cloves, chopped

1 pound ground lamb (from leg)

1 tablespoon curry powder

1/2 teaspoon ground cinnamon

Sea salt and freshly ground black pepper

CUCUMBER-MINT SOUR CREAM
1/2 medium cucumber, peeled, seeded, and diced

1/4 cup chopped fresh mint, plus leaves for garnish

1/3 cup sour cream

Juice from 2 limes

RADICCHIO CUPS
8 radicchio leaves

minted lamb in cucumber boats with marinated red onions

PROTEIN, HEALTHY FATS, VEGETABLES

DETOX, LEVEL 1, LEVEL 2

VEGETABLES

1 red onion, sliced paper-thin

Juice from 6 limes

Sea salt

6 small pickling cucumbers, such as Kirby

MINTED LAMB

2 tablespoons olive oil

3 serrano chiles, seeded and finely chopped (see Note, page 39)

1 tablespoon minced fresh ginger

4 garlic cloves, chopped

3/4 pound ground lamb (from leg)

1 tablespoon Thai fish sauce (nam pla; optional)

Freshly ground black pepper

3 tablespoons chopped fresh mint

Juice from 2 limes

For the vegetables: Place the onion in a nonreactive bowl with the lime juice and a pinch of salt. Let stand for a few hours.

Cut the cucumbers in half lengthwise. Scoop out a good portion of the center with a spoon or a melon baller, creating a boat shape to hold the lamb filling. (I like the skin of unwaxed cucumbers, so I leave it on. If you don't like it, peel the skin off before you cut the cucumber.) Place in refrigerator.

For the lamb: Heat a sauté pan over medium heat. Add the oil, then the chiles. Cook for 2 to 3 minutes. Add the ginger and garlic and cook until golden brown, about 1 minute. Add the lamb and brown over medium-high heat, seasoning with the fish sauce, if using, and pepper. When the meat is cooked through, about 10 minutes, remove from the heat and toss with the mint and lime juice.

Fill the cucumber boats with the minted lamb and top with marinated onion.   SERVES 8

angel eggs with crème fraîche and caviar

PROTEIN, HEALTHY FATS, VEGETABLES

DETOX, LEVEL 1, LEVEL 2

Slice the eggs in half lengthwise, being careful not to tear the whites. Remove the yolks and press through a fine sieve or finely chop. In a small bowl, mix the yolks with the crème fraîche and season with salt and pepper. Spoon a little of the yolk mixture into each egg half and garnish with a dollop of caviar and a sprinkle of chives. Serve immediately.　MAKES 16

8 large eggs, hard-boiled and peeled

1/4 cup crème fraîche (page 149) or sour cream

Sea salt and freshly ground black pepper

1/2 ounce caviar

2 tablespoons finely minced fresh chives

deviled eggs

PROTEIN, HEALTHY FATS, VEGETABLES

DETOX, LEVEL 1, LEVEL 2

Put the eggs in a medium saucepan and cover with cold water. Place over medium-high heat and bring to a boil. Reduce the heat a little until the water reaches a low boil and cook for 15 minutes.

Drain and run the eggs under cold water. Set aside to let the eggs cool.

When cooled, peel the eggs. Slice the eggs in half lengthwise. Place all the yolks in a small mixing bowl. Add the mayonnaise, mustard, if using, and salt and pepper to taste. Mash together with a fork until smooth and well combined.

Arrange the egg whites on a platter with the cavity side up. Spoon some of the filling into each hole until all are filled. Top with chopped chives and a sprinkle of paprika. Refrigerate until ready to serve.　MAKES 12

6 large eggs

1 to 2 tablespoons mayonnaise

1/4 teaspoon dry mustard (optional)

Sea salt and freshly ground black pepper

1 bunch chives, finely chopped

Paprika

clams gratin with pancetta and arugula

PROTEIN, HEALTHY FATS, VEGETABLES

LEVEL 1, LEVEL 2

Extra virgin olive oil

1 garlic clove, smashed

16 to 18 cherrystone
clams, or other fresh
clams, scrubbed

$^1/_2$ cup dry white wine

Sea salt and freshly
ground black pepper

1 cup arugula

$^1/_4$ cup pancetta or
bacon, cooked until
crispy, crumbled

Freshly grated
Parmesan cheese,
for garnish

Preheat the boiler.

In a large sauté pan over medium-high heat, warm enough olive oil to coat the pan. Add the garlic and allow it to brown. Add the clams and toss in the oil to coat. Add the wine and season with salt and pepper. Cover the pan and cook until the clams open. When they are opened, remove them from the heat immediately and allow to cool. (Discard any clams that do not open.) When the clams are cool enough to handle, discard the top half of the shells. Reserve the clam broth. Place the clams in their shells on a baking sheet.

Wilt the arugula in a hot sauté pan with a bit of olive oil. Remove from the heat to cool. Finely chop the arugula.

Spoon a little of the clam broth over the top of the clams and sprinkle with the pancetta, arugula, and Parmesan cheese. Place under the broiler for 3 minutes. Serve immediately.   MAKES 16

saffron mussels with red pepper rouille

PROTEIN, HEALTHY FATS, VEGETABLES

LEVEL 1, LEVEL 2

In a large sauté pan over medium heat, add enough olive oil to cover the bottom of the pan. Add the shallots and mussels. Gently toss to coat with oil. Add the saffron and wine, cover, and cook until the mussels open, 3 to 4 minutes. (Discard any mussels that do not open.) Add the butter to the pan and season to taste with salt and pepper. Allow to slightly cool. When cool enough to handle, discard the top half of each shell and serve the mussels on the half shell with a dollop of rouille and a sprig of fresh fennel leaf. MAKES 16

Olive oil

2 tablespoons minced shallots

1 pound (about 16) mussels, scrubbed

1/4 teaspoon saffron threads

1 cup dry white wine

1 tablespoon unsalted butter

Sea salt and freshly ground black pepper

3/4 cup Red Pepper Rouille (page 152)

Fresh fennel leaves

grilled scallops wrapped in prosciutto with basil-parsley pesto

PROTEIN, HEALTHY FATS, VEGETABLES

LEVEL 1, LEVEL 2

Preheat grill to high.

Loosely wrap each scallop with ½ piece prosciutto. Season with salt and pepper, drizzle with olive oil, and secure on a skewer.

Grill the wrapped scallops until evenly browned, 2 to 3 minutes on each side. Remove from the grill and serve with a small dollop of pesto. MAKES 16

4 large sea scallops, quartered, or 16 smaller scallops

8 thin slices prosciutto, cut in half

Sea salt and freshly ground black pepper

Extra virgin olive oil

16 wooden skewers, soaked in water

1 cup Basil-Parsley Pesto (page 150)

red hot singing scallops

PROTEIN, HEALTHY FATS, VEGETABLES

DETOX, LEVEL 1, LEVEL 2

18 small scallops, in the shell (if available)

¹/₄ cup mayonnaise

8 to 10 dashes hot pepper sauce, such as Cholula

1 tablespoon finely chopped flat-leaf parsley

Preheat the broiler.

Open the scallops and discard the top shells. Arrange in a single layer on a baking sheet. In a small bowl, combine the mayonnaise with the hot sauce to reach your desired level of spice. Place a small dollop on each scallop. Sprinkle with a tiny bit of parsley.

Broil for about 3 minutes, or until the scallops begin to bubble. Serve immediately.   MAKES 18

sweet shrimp with hot green chutney

PROTEIN, HEALTHY FATS, VEGETABLES
LEVEL 1, LEVEL 2

For the chutney: In a medium saucepan over medium heat, add the olive oil, onion, and ginger. Cook until the onion is soft, 5 to 6 minutes, stirring occasionally. Add the vinegar and All Natural SomerSweet. Simmer for 2 minutes. Remove from the heat and allow to cool. When cool, add the chiles and herbs. Adjust the seasoning with salt and pepper. Set aside to serve with the shrimp.

For the shrimp: Season the shrimp with salt and pepper. In a medium sauté pan over medium heat, add a tablespoon of olive oil. Add the shrimp, gently searing on both sides. Add the wine. Reduce the heat and cover. Cook until the shrimp are just cooked through, about 3 minutes, depending upon their size. Remove from the heat, and place the shrimp on a plate.

Serve the shrimp with the dipping sauce.　MAKES 16

HOT GREEN CHUTNEY

1 tablespoon extra virgin olive oil

1/2 yellow onion, finely diced

2 tablespoons finely minced fresh ginger

1/4 cup rice vinegar

1/2 teaspoon All Natural SomerSweet, or 2 teaspoons sugar

1 red jalapeño chile, finely minced (see Note, page 39)

1 serrano chile, finely minced

1/2 cup chopped fresh cilantro

1/4 cup chopped fresh basil

1/4 cup chopped fresh mint

Sea salt and freshly ground black pepper

SHRIMP

16 large raw shrimp, peeled and deveined, tails left on

Sea salt and freshly ground black pepper

Extra virgin olive oil

2 cups dry white wine

rock shrimp salad on cucumber rounds

PROTEIN, HEALTHY FATS, VEGETABLES

DETOX, LEVEL 1, LEVEL 2

1 tablespoon extra
    virgin olive oil

1 garlic clove, smashed

$\frac{1}{2}$ pound rock shrimp,
    cleaned (see Note,
    page 82)

$\frac{1}{2}$ cup mayonnaise

$\frac{1}{4}$ cup sour cream

$\frac{1}{2}$ red bell pepper,
    seeded and finely
    diced

$\frac{1}{2}$ red onion, finely
    diced

2 scallions, white and
    some green parts,
    finely diced

Tabasco sauce

Sea salt and freshly
    ground black pepper

Juice from 1 lemon

1 medium cucumber

In a medium sauté pan over medium heat, add the olive oil and garlic. As the garlic becomes golden brown, add the shrimp and cook until just done, 3 to 4 minutes. Remove from the heat and chill.

In a mixing bowl, combine the mayonnaise, sour cream, red pepper, onion, scallions, and a dash of Tabasco. Chop half the shrimp and leave the other half whole, then add all the shrimp to the salad ingredients and mix well. Adjust the seasoning with salt, pepper, and lemon juice. Set aside.

Peel the cucumber in 4 strips lengthwise to create a wide scoring effect, then slice into ½-inch rounds. Carefully scoop out some of the seeds to create a small indentation (without scooping all the way through) to cradle the filling. Fill each cucumber slice with a scoop of shrimp salad and serve immediately. MAKES ABOUT 16 ROUNDS

tuna tartare with chile-ginger vinaigrette on pappadam chips

PROTEIN, HEALTHY FATS, VEGETABLES, INSULIN TRIGGERS

LEVEL 2

Tear the pappadams into 16 chip-size pieces. Pour oil into a deep, heavy pot until one-third full. Heat on high until the temperature reaches 375°F. Fry the pappadams a few pieces at a time until they bubble and float. Remove and drain on paper towels. Set aside.

Clean and dice the tuna. Place in a small mixing bowl with the remaining ingredients except the cilantro, and mix well. Adjust the seasoning to taste. Spoon the tuna mixture onto a chip, garnish with the cilantro, and serve immediately. MAKES 16

4 pieces Indian pappadam flatbread

Coconut or grapeseed oil

1 pound sushi-grade ahi tuna

1 tablespoon finely minced fresh ginger

1/2 jalapeño or serrano chile, finely minced (see Note, page 39)

2 teaspoons soy sauce

1 teaspoon sesame oil

1 teaspoon rice vinegar

Juice from 1/2 lime

Sea salt and freshly ground black pepper

1 scallion, green parts only, finely chopped

Cilantro leaves, for garnish

seared tuna with cilantro-orange sauce

PROTEIN, HEALTHY FATS, VEGETABLES,
CARBOHYDRATES, FRUIT

LEVEL 2

8 ounces ahi tuna, cut
into about 16 bite-
size cubes

Sea salt and freshly
ground black pepper

Extra virgin olive oil

Dash of soy sauce

Juice from $\frac{1}{2}$ lime

Cilantro-Orange Sauce
(recipe follows)

Season the tuna with salt and pepper. Heat a light coating of olive oil in a sauté pan over medium-high heat, then sear the tuna on all sides until golden brown on the outside but rare in the center. Remove from the heat and drizzle with soy sauce and lime juice. Place on a platter with toothpicks and serve with cilantro-orange sauce for dipping.

MAKES ABOUT 16 CUBES

cilantro-orange sauce

HEALTHY FATS, VEGETABLES, CARBOHYDRATES, FRUIT

LEVEL 2

$\frac{1}{2}$ cup orange juice

1 tablespoon miso paste

2 tablespoons chopped fresh cilantro

2 tablespoons chopped scallions

Juice from 1 lime

$\frac{1}{2}$ cup extra virgin olive oil

Combine all the ingredients in a blender and puree until smooth. MAKES 1 CUP

grilled vegetable antipasto

HEALTHY FATS, VEGETABLES

DETOX, LEVEL 1, LEVEL 2

Preheat the grill or grill pan.

Place the radicchio, fennel, red peppers, eggplant, baby onions, red onions, and rosemary in a large bowl. Toss with the olive oil and season with salt and pepper. Place the vegetables on the hot grill, turning several times and removing once grill marks have appeared. The vegetables are best-tasting when they are tender but still slightly crisp. Arrange them on a platter.

Roughly chop the candied tomatoes and add to the platter. Squeeze the cloves of baked garlic into a small bowl, then spread evenly over the vegetables. Drizzle with fresh-squeezed lemon and balsamic vinegar. SERVES 8

2 heads radicchio, quartered

2 fennel bulbs, thinly sliced

3 red bell peppers, seeded and cut into chunky strips

1 large eggplant, sliced into $1/2$-inch rounds

1 pound baby onions

2 red onions, quartered

8 long sprigs fresh rosemary

$1/2$ cup extra virgin olive oil

Sea salt and freshly ground black pepper

8 Candied Tomatoes (page 174)

8 heads Baked Garlic (page 166)

8 lemon wedges

Balsamic vinegar, for garnish

baba ghanoush

HEALTHY FATS, VEGETABLES, CARBOHYDRATES

LEVEL 1, LEVEL 2

1 large eggplant

Juice from 1 lemon

3 garlic cloves, chopped

5 to 8 dashes Tabasco sauce

3 tablespoons tahini

Place the eggplant on a prepared grill over medium heat, turning occasionally, until blackened and soft on all sides, about 30 minutes. (Or you can roast the eggplant in the oven on a baking sheet, turning often until the eggplant is roasted on all sides.)

Remove the eggplant from the heat. Immediately place it in a paper bag, close the bag, and let the eggplant steam for about 30 minutes. Remove the eggplant from the bag, peel off the skin and stem, and place the meat in a food processor. Add the remaining ingredients, puree, and adjust seasonings to taste.   MAKES 1$\frac{1}{2}$ CUPS

NOTE Serve with crudités or whole wheat pita triangles.

hummus

HEALTHY FATS, VEGETABLES, CARBOHYDRATES
LEVEL 1, LEVEL 2

In a food processor or blender, puree the garbanzos with the garlic, lemon juice, cayenne, salt, pepper, and tahini until smooth. Adjust seasoning to taste. Garnish with a sprig of parsley, a sprinkle of cayenne, and pine nuts, if desired.   SERVES 4

NOTE Serve with crudités or whole wheat pita triangles.

4 cups cooked or canned garbanzo beans (chickpeas)

3 garlic cloves

4 tablespoons lemon juice

Dash of cayenne

Sea salt and freshly ground black pepper

2 tablespoons tahini

1 sprig flat-leaf parsley

1/4 cup toasted pine nuts (optional)

cannellini bean dip

HEALTHY FATS, VEGETABLES, CARBOHYDRATES
LEVEL 1, LEVEL 2

Place all the ingredients except the pine nuts in a food processor or blender. Puree until smooth. Adjust seasonings to taste, and add more lemon juice if desired. Garnish with the pine nuts.   MAKES 1 1/2 CUPS

NOTE Serve with crudités or whole wheat pita triangles.

3 cups cooked cannellini beans (or any other white beans)

1 garlic clove

Juice from 1 lemon

2 tablespoons chopped fresh sage or flat-leaf parsley

Sea salt and freshly ground black pepper

2 tablespoons extra virgin olive oil

1/4 cup toasted pine nuts

roasted red peppers and grilled bread

HEALTHY FATS, VEGETABLES, CARBOHYDRATES

LEVEL 1, LEVEL 2

ROASTED RED
PEPPERS

4 red bell peppers

GRILLED BREAD

4 slices of whole-grain
bread

4 whole garlic cloves
(1 per slice of bread)

1 tablespoon extra
virgin olive oil

For the roasted peppers: Place the whole peppers on a prepared hot grill or an open flame and char on all sides until the skins are black and bubbling. Immediately put the roasted peppers into a paper bag and close. Let the peppers steam in the bag for 15 minutes. (This steaming process will make the peeling easier.)

Remove the peppers from the bag and pull the stems off. Break the peppers apart and discard the seeds. The charred skins will peel off easily. (I find it's faster to seed and peel the peppers under cool running water.) Break into strips and arrange on a platter.

For the grilled bread: Grill the bread slices over high heat, turning when nicely toasted on each side. While still warm, rub the bread slices with garlic. Drizzle with oil. Serve each slice with a strip of the roasted red pepper.   SERVES 4

candied tomato tart

HEALTHY FATS, VEGETABLES, INSULIN TRIGGERS

LEVEL 2

5 or 6 sheets phyllo
dough

¼ cup olive oil

24 Candied Tomatoes
(page 174)

Preheat the oven to 350°F. Thaw the phyllo dough.

Put one layer of phyllo on a cookie sheet and brush lightly with olive oil. Fold in the ends to create an edge for a 9 × 6-inch tart, securing with a little more olive oil (or make any shape or size desired by cutting the phyllo dough). Continue with another sheet of phyllo, brushing with oil and creating an edge. After about five or six layers, you should have a nice-looking ruffled edge and a center area to fill with the tomatoes.

Start on the outside edge and arrange the tomato halves, fanning them together in a pattern like the petals of a flower. Bake for 25 minutes, or until the phyllo is brown on the edges.

Cut the tart into six squares and serve hot or at room temperature.

MAKES 6 APPETIZERS, OR 3 ENTRÉES WITH A GREEN SALAD

whole wheat popovers

PROTEIN, HEALTHY FATS, CARBOHYDRATES, INSULIN TRIGGERS

LEVEL 2

1 cup nonfat milk

1 tablespoon melted
unsalted butter

1 cup whole wheat
pastry flour

¼ teaspoon sea salt

2 large eggs

Preheat the oven to 450°F. Butter an 8-cup popover pan.

In a large bowl, beat the milk, butter, flour, and salt together until smooth. Add the eggs, one at a time, being careful not to overbeat. Fill the popover or muffin cups three-fourths full. Bake for 15 minutes. Without opening the oven door, turn the heat down to 350°F and bake an additional 20 minutes. Serve immediately. MAKES 8 POPOVERS

flourless cheese soufflé

2 tablespoons unsalted
  butter, softened

6 large eggs, separated

Pinch of cayenne

$1/2$ teaspoon freshly
  grated nutmeg

Sea salt and freshly
  ground black pepper

4 ounces cream cheese,
  softened

$1^1/2$ cups finely grated
  Gruyère or Swiss
  cheese

PROTEIN, HEALTHY FATS
DETOX, LEVEL 1, LEVEL 2

Preheat the oven to 425°F. Coat a 6-cup soufflé dish with butter.

In a mixing bowl, combine the egg yolks, cayenne, nutmeg, salt, and pepper. Beat with a wire whisk until light and fluffy. Add the cream cheese and grated cheese and whisk until well combined and smooth.

In another bowl, beat the egg whites until somewhat stiff peaks form. Fold the egg whites into the cheese mixture. Spoon into the greased dish and place on a baking sheet.

Bake for 10 minutes. Reduce the heat to 400°F and bake an additional 15 minutes. Serve immediately. SERVES 4

chicken and roasted vegetable sandwiches

PROTEIN, HEALTHY FATS, VEGETABLES

DETOX, LEVEL 1, LEVEL 2

Preheat the oven to 425°F.

For the vegetables: Place the eggplant, mushrooms, zucchini, onions, and tomatoes on baking sheets. In a small bowl, combine the olive oil, vinegar, thyme, salt, pepper, and red pepper flakes. Lightly brush on the vegetables and bake, removing the vegetables as they each become golden brown (the zucchini and eggplant in about 15 minutes, then the mushrooms and onions; the tomatoes will take up to 45 minutes).

For the chicken breasts: Pound each breast with a mallet until about ⅓ inch thick. Season with rosemary, salt, and pepper. Heat a large skillet over medium-high heat. Add a little olive oil and sauté the chicken on each side until nicely browned and just cooked through, about 5 minutes.

For the sandwiches: On a baking sheet, using the eggplant as the "bread," layer a chicken piece, then slices of mozzarella, tomato, zucchini, 2 mushrooms, and an onion slice, ending with another eggplant slice. (You may have to trim the chicken and zucchini to fit the shape of the eggplant slices.) Secure the sandwiches with toothpicks or sprigs of rosemary, if using.

Heat sandwiches in oven for 5 minutes at 425°F, or until the mozzarella has melted. MAKES 4 SANDWICHES

ROASTED VEGETABLES

1 large eggplant, cut lengthwise into 8 slices, about ⅓ inch thick

Caps of 8 large shiitake mushrooms

3 medium zucchini, cut lengthwise into ¼-inch slices

2 red onions, cut into ¼-inch slices

8 ripe medium tomatoes, sliced in half crosswise

3 tablespoons olive oil

2 teaspoons balsamic vinegar

½ teaspoon chopped fresh thyme leaves

Sea salt and freshly ground black pepper

¼ teaspoon red pepper flakes

CHICKEN BREASTS

Two 6-ounce skinless and boneless chicken breasts, separated into halves

2 teaspoons dried rosemary

Sea salt and freshly ground black pepper

2 tablespoons olive oil

SANDWICHES

½ pound fresh mozzarella, cut into ¼-inch slices

Sprigs of fresh rosemary (optional)

pita sandwiches with vegetables and yogurt cheese

VEGETABLES, CARBOHYDRATES

LEVEL 1, LEVEL 2

1 cup plain nonfat yogurt

2 whole wheat pitas

4 Roasted Red Peppers (page 134) or jarred roasted peppers in water

2 slices sweet onion

1/2 medium cucumber, thinly sliced

A few arugula leaves or red leaf lettuce

Balsamic vinegar

1/4 teaspoon dried oregano

Sea salt and freshly ground black pepper

Line a fine strainer with cheesecloth. Place the yogurt in the strainer with a bowl underneath to catch the liquid. Refrigerate overnight. Most of the moisture will drain out of the yogurt, creating a soft, delicious cheese. Refrigerate. (Makes about ¾ cup.)

Slice one edge off the pita breads to make a pouch with an opening. Toast the pitas, then fill with the peppers, onion, cucumber, and arugula.

Spoon some of the yogurt cheese on the vegetables and drizzle balsamic vinegar over it. Then sprinkle with the oregano, salt, and pepper and serve.   SERVES 2

b.l.t. in lettuce cups

PROTEIN, HEALTHY FATS, VEGETABLES

DETOX, LEVEL 1, LEVEL 2

6 bacon slices

1 head iceberg lettuce

3 to 4 tablespoons mayonnaise

2 ripe medium tomatoes, chopped

Place a small skillet over medium-high heat. Add the bacon and fry until golden brown, about 5 minutes. Turn off the heat, then remove the bacon and drain on paper towels. When cooled, crumble into small pieces.

Make 6 lettuce "cups" by carefully peeling the leaves off of the head, trying to keep them whole. Chop the remaining lettuce into thin strips.

Arrange 3 lettuce cups on each plate. Spread as much mayonnaise as you like onto each. Place a small handful of chopped lettuce into each cup. Add the chopped tomatoes, evenly dividing them among the lettuce cups. Top with the crumbled bacon. Fold up and eat like a taco.   SERVES 2

veggie wrap

VEGETABLES, CARBOHYDRATES
DETOX, LEVEL 1, LEVEL 2

Preheat the oven to 350°F.

Salt the eggplant and the zucchini slices on both sides and place in a colander to let the excess water drain. Rinse and pat dry. Place the slices in a single layer on cookie sheets. Bake for approximately 20 minutes. Remove any smaller pieces as they become brown, so as not to burn any of the slices.

Lay the lavash or tortilla flat on a chopping block. Spread the ricotta cheese in a thin layer over each entire piece. Season with salt and pepper. Place the eggplant in a single layer over the ricotta. Then place a single layer of the zucchini. Place the peppers in a single row down the middle. Top with a lettuce leaf. Roll up the bread or tortilla and secure with a toothpick (or use a tiny bit of water to "glue" the tortilla to the other side). Slice on the diagonal and serve. SERVES 4

Sea salt

1 large eggplant, sliced paper-thin

2 medium zucchini, sliced paper-thin

4 pieces whole wheat lavash bread, or 4 whole wheat fat-free tortillas

1 cup nonfat ricotta cheese

Freshly ground black pepper

2 Roasted Red Peppers (page 134) or jarred roasted peppers in water

4 red leaf lettuce leaves

dressings, sauces, and pesto

the toppers

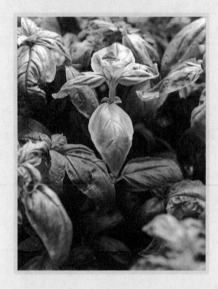

A drizzle, a puddle, a toss, a dollop . . . sometimes it's the extra special accessory to the food that takes it from good to spectacular. Many of the sauces or dressings in this recipe bible are already attached to their featured recipes, but these gems are placed here so you can use them at will with any of your favorite dishes.

The base for most of my salad dressings is a great quality oil. I was introduced to the Malibu Olive Company at a farmers' market and have fallen deeply in love with their Romanelli Quattro Blend extra virgin olive oil. Not only a healthy fat with essential omega-3 oils, it's great for your skin, hair, heart, organs, cell reproduction, and—did I mention making everything taste incredible?

If you are used to bottled dressing, it takes a quick shift in thinking to decide to make your own. We are talking about less than 5 minutes for most of these dressings. Wait until you see how easy it is to make Blue Cheese Dip (page 146). Just sour cream, blue cheese crumbles, salt and pepper, and a little red wine vinegar. Done!

This whole recipe section is worth reading for the Basil-Parsley Pesto (page 150) alone. It's the best pesto recipe I have ever used and it gets a lot of action in my house when my garden basil sprouts to its full glory. I make jars and jars of it, then freeze it so I have a supply at all times. Blanching the herbs first keeps their bright green pop of color. They are delicious and bursting with health-saving antioxidants. If you are planning to freeze the pesto, hold the cheese and add it at the last minute when the pesto is thawed and ready to enjoy. I use pesto liberally in soups, on meats, in salads, and tossed into quinoa or brown rice pasta.

Also not to be missed, my Homemade Mayonnaise (page 148); it's light and delicious with just the right tang of citrus. My daughter-in-law, Caroline, makes it every year to serve at our family's Crab Lunch with warm, just-steamed Dungeness crab. I have switched to grapeseed oil for this recipe. It's another of the healthy oils and it has a neutral flavor that keeps the mayonnaise light and fresh.

Top that.

garlic vinaigrette

HEALTHY FATS, VEGETABLES

DETOX, LEVEL 1, LEVEL 2

2 to 3 garlic cloves, pressed

Juice from 1 lemon

Sea salt and freshly ground black pepper

¼ cup extra virgin olive oil

Mix the garlic, lemon juice, salt, and pepper in a small bowl. Add the olive oil in a slow stream, whisking constantly until combined.

Store in an airtight container in the refrigerator for 2 to 3 weeks. MAKES ¼ CUP

champagne mustard vinaigrette

HEALTHY FATS, VEGETABLES

DETOX, LEVEL 1, LEVEL 2

2 shallots, finely minced

2 tablespoons Dijon mustard

4 tablespoons Champagne vinegar

1 cup extra virgin olive oil

Juice from ¼ lemon

Sea salt and freshly ground black pepper

In a medium bowl, combine the shallots, mustard, and vinegar. Whisk in the olive oil until completely smooth. Add the lemon juice and season to taste with salt and pepper.

Store in an airtight container in the refrigerator for 2 to 3 weeks. MAKES ABOUT 1 CUP

balsamic vinaigrette

HEALTHY FATS

DETOX, LEVEL 1, LEVEL 2

    gf df ef v vg

Place the vinegar in a small bowl and whisk in salt and pepper to taste. Add the olive oil in a slow stream, whisking constantly until the oil is emulsified. For a tangier dressing, add more balsamic vinegar.

Store in an airtight container in the refrigerator for 2 to 3 weeks. MAKES ABOUT $^1\!/_2$ CUP

2 tablespoons balsamic vinegar

Sea salt and freshly ground black pepper

6 tablespoons extra virgin olive oil

red wine vinaigrette

HEALTHY FATS

DETOX, LEVEL 1, LEVEL 2

     gf df ef v vg

Combine the vinegar, oregano, lemon juice, and salt and pepper to taste in a small bowl. Add the olive oil in a slow stream, whisking constantly until the oil is emulsified.

Store in an airtight container in the refrigerator for 2 to 3 weeks. MAKES ABOUT 1 CUP

$^1\!/_2$ cup red wine vinegar

$^1\!/_2$ teaspoon dried oregano

$^1\!/_2$ teaspoon fresh lemon juice

$^1\!/_8$ teaspoon sea salt

$^1\!/_8$ teaspoon freshly ground black pepper

$^1\!/_3$ cup extra virgin olive oil

herb vinaigrette

HEALTHY FATS, VEGETABLES
DETOX, LEVEL 1, LEVEL 2

2 tablespoons red wine vinegar

1 garlic clove, pressed

2 teaspoons whole-grain mustard

1 teaspoon dried dill weed

1 teaspoon dried thyme

Sea salt and freshly ground black pepper

6 tablespoons extra virgin olive oil

In a small bowl, whisk together all the ingredients except the olive oil. Add the oil in a slow stream, whisking constantly until the oil is emulsified. For a tangier dressing, add more vinegar.

Store in an airtight container in the refrigerator for 2 to 3 weeks. MAKES ABOUT ³/₄ CUP

lemon tarragon vinaigrette

HEALTHY FATS
DETOX, LEVEL 1, LEVEL 2

¹/₂ cup tarragon vinegar

¹/₂ teaspoon chopped fresh thyme

1 teaspoon chopped fresh oregano

1 teaspoon fresh lemon juice

¹/₂ teaspoon grated lemon zest

¹/₃ cup extra virgin olive oil

¹/₄ teaspoon sea salt

¹/₈ teaspoon freshly ground black pepper

In a small bowl, whisk together the vinegar, herbs, lemon juice, zest, and salt and pepper. Add the olive oil in a slow stream, whisking constantly until the oil is emulsified. Adjust the seasonings.

Store in an airtight container in the refrigerator for 2 to 3 weeks. MAKES 1 CUP

french dressing

HEALTHY FATS

DETOX, LEVEL 1, LEVEL 2

Place the salt, pepper, mustard, and vinegar in a small bowl and whisk to combine. Add the olive oil in a slow, steady stream, whisking constantly until the oil is emulsified. Add the hot pepper oil while continuing to whisk. Adjust seasonings to taste.

Store in an airtight container in the refrigerator for 2 to 3 weeks. MAKES ABOUT ½ CUP

Sea salt and freshly ground black pepper

1 teaspoon dry mustard

2 tablespoons tarragon or white wine vinegar

½ cup extra virgin olive oil

1 teaspoon hot pepper oil

blue cheese vinaigrette

HEALTHY FATS

DETOX, LEVEL 1, LEVEL 2

Place the vinegar in a small bowl and whisk in salt and pepper to taste. Add the olive oil in a slow stream, constantly whisking until the oil is emulsified. Add the blue cheese to the vinaigrette and stir until combined.

Store in an airtight container in the refrigerator for up to 1 week. MAKES ABOUT ¾ CUP

2 tablespoons balsamic vinegar

Sea salt and freshly ground black pepper

6 tablespoons extra virgin olive oil

6 ounces blue cheese (preferably Roquefort), crumbled

blue cheese dip

HEALTHY FATS

DETOX, LEVEL 1, LEVEL 2

3/4 cup sour cream

2 tablespoons red wine vinegar

4 ounces blue cheese (preferably Maytag or Roquefort), crumbled

Sea salt and freshly ground black pepper

Combine all the ingredients in a bowl, mashing the cheese with a fork until well combined. If the dressing is too thick, add a little more vinegar.

Store in an airtight container in the refrigerator for up to 1 week. MAKES ABOUT 1 1/2 CUPS

green goddess dressing

HEALTHY FATS, VEGETABLES

DETOX, LEVEL 1, LEVEL 2

4 scallions, white and green parts, thinly sliced

1 1/2 cups mayonnaise

Juice from 2 limes (about 1/4 cup)

Trim the ends off the scallions. Roughly chop the white and green parts and place in a food processor or blender. Chop until coarsely ground. Add the mayonnaise and lime juice, and puree until smooth.

Store in an airtight container in the refrigerator for up to 1 week. MAKES ABOUT 1 1/2 CUPS

pink goddess salad dressing

PROTEIN, HEALTHY FATS

DETOX, LEVEL 1, LEVEL 2

Combine the vinegar, lemon juice, mayonnaise, and All Natural SomerSweet in a small bowl. Drizzle in the olive oil, whisking constantly, until mixture is creamy. Add the salt and pepper.

Store in an airtight container in the refrigerator for up to 1 week.

MAKES 1¼ CUPS

FOR LEVEL 2   For a Level 2 dressing, omit the red wine vinegar and mayonnaise, and use one 5-ounce container of fresh raspberries. Place all the ingredients in a food processor or blender and pulse until smooth.

⅓ cup red wine vinegar

2 teaspoons fresh lemon juice

3 tablespoons mayonnaise

1½ teaspoons All Natural SomerSweet

⅔ cup extra virgin olive oil

¼ teaspoon sea salt

⅛ teaspoon freshly ground black pepper

roasted red pepper vinaigrette

HEALTHY FATS, VEGETABLES

DETOX, LEVEL 1, LEVEL 2

    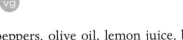

Place the roasted peppers, olive oil, lemon juice, basil, oregano, and garlic in the blender. Puree until smooth. Season to taste with salt and pepper.

Store in an airtight container in the refrigerator for 1 to 2 weeks.   MAKES ABOUT 1 CUP

1 cup Roasted Red Peppers (page 134) or jarred roasted peppers in water

¼ cup extra virgin olive oil

1 tablespoon fresh lemon juice

4 fresh basil leaves, chopped

1 teaspoon dried oregano

1 teaspoon minced fresh garlic

Sea salt and freshly ground black pepper

homemade mayonnaise

2 large organic eggs

1 teaspoon red wine vinegar

Juice from 1/2 lemon

1/2 teaspoon sea salt

1/4 teaspoon ground white pepper

Dash of Tabasco sauce

Dash of Worcestershire sauce (see Note, page 45)

1 cup grapeseed or light olive oil

Combine all the ingredients except the oil in a bowl. Add the oil very gradually in a thin stream, whisking constantly until the mayonnaise emulsifies. Adjust the seasonings to taste. (This can also be prepared in a blender or food processor.)

Store in an airtight container in the refrigerator for up to 1 week.

MAKES 1 1/2 CUPS

lemon-dill mayonnaise

1 recipe Homemade Mayonnaise (above) or prepared mayonnaise

Juice from 1 lemon

1 tablespoon finely chopped fresh dill or 2 teaspoons dried dill weed

Freshly ground black pepper

Prepare the mayonnaise as above, adding additional lemon juice, the dill, and black pepper.

Store in an airtight container in the refrigerator for up to 1 week.

MAKES ABOUT 1/2 CUP

crème fraîche

HEALTHY FATS

DETOX, LEVEL 1, LEVEL 2

1 cup sour cream

1 cup heavy cream

Combine the ingredients in a bowl until slightly thickened. Let sit out at room temperature for several hours to thicken and sour a bit.

Store in an airtight container in the refrigerator for up to 1 week.

MAKES ABOUT 1 CUP

artichoke pesto

HEALTHY FATS, VEGETABLES

DETOX, LEVEL 1, LEVEL 2

4 artichoke bottoms, freshly steamed or canned in water

6 garlic cloves, chopped

1/2 cup mayonnaise

1/2 cup freshly grated Parmesan cheese

4 scallions, white and green parts, sliced

2 teaspoons fresh lemon juice

1/2 cup extra virgin olive oil

Sea salt and freshly ground black pepper

Place all the ingredients in a food processor and pulse until smooth. Season with salt and pepper to taste.

Store in an airtight container in the refrigerator for up to 2 weeks.   MAKES ABOUT 3 CUPS

basil-parsley pesto

HEALTHY FATS, VEGETABLES, CARBOHYDRATES
DETOX, LEVEL 1, LEVEL 2

2 cups basil leaves,
loosely packed

1/2 cup flat-leaf parsley,
loosely packed

1/2 cup freshly grated
Parmesan cheese

1/4 cup toasted pine
nuts (omit for Detox)

3/4 cup extra virgin
olive oil

1 garlic clove, minced

1/2 teaspoon sea salt

Freshly ground black
pepper

Set aside a small bowl filled with ice and water. Bring a small pot of water to a boil and add the basil leaves for 30 seconds to soften. Remove immediately and plunge the leaves into the ice water. After 30 to 60 seconds, remove the leaves from the ice bath, squeeze out excess water, and place into a blender or food processor. Add the remaining ingredients and puree until smooth.

Store in an airtight container in the refrigerator for up to 2 weeks. For information on freezing, see page 141.   MAKES ABOUT 1 CUP

parsley pesto

HEALTHY FATS, VEGETABLES
DETOX, LEVEL 1, LEVEL 2

1/2 bunch flat-leaf
parsley, leaves only

1 bunch fresh tarragon,
leaves only

1/4 cup freshly grated
Parmesan cheese

1 garlic clove, minced

1 1/2 cups extra virgin
olive oil

Juice of 1 lemon

Place all the ingredients except the lemon juice into a blender or food processor and blend until smooth. Add the lemon juice at the very end to prevent discoloration of the herbs.

Store in an airtight container in the refrigerator for up to 2 weeks. For information on freezing, see page 141.   MAKES ABOUT 1 CUP

sun-dried tomato pesto

HEALTHY FATS, VEGETABLES

DETOX, LEVEL 1, LEVEL 2

    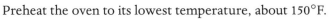

12 Roma (plum) tomatoes, thinly sliced

Sea salt and freshly ground black pepper

1/4 cup extra virgin olive oil, plus more for sprinkling

Preheat the oven to its lowest temperature, about 150°F.

Lay the tomato slices on baking sheets. Sprinkle them with salt and pepper and a little olive oil. Place on center rack of the oven. Let the tomatoes dry for about 3 hours. They should feel dry to the touch but not dried out. Rotate the baking sheets every now and then so the tomatoes cook evenly.

Remove the tomatoes from the oven and place them in a blender or food processor. Add the olive oil and pulse until roughly pureed.

Store in an airtight container in the refrigerator for up to 2 weeks.   MAKES 1 1/2 CUPS

mint-cilantro pesto

HEALTHY FATS, VEGETABLES, CARBOHYDRATES

DETOX, LEVEL 1, LEVEL 2

1/2 bunch fresh cilantro, leaves removed

1/2 bunch fresh mint, leaves removed

2 tablespoons toasted pine nuts (omit for Detox)

1/4 cup extra virgin olive oil

Sea salt and freshly ground black pepper

Juice from 1/2 lemon

Place all the ingredients except the lemon juice into a blender or food processor and puree until smooth. Add the lemon juice and pulse to combine. Adjust the seasonings to taste.

Store in an airtight container in the refrigerator for up to 2 weeks.   MAKES ABOUT 1 CUP

red pepper rouille

HEALTHY FATS, VEGETABLES

DETOX, LEVEL 1, LEVEL 2

1 Roasted Red Pepper
(page 134), or
1 jarred roasted
pepper in water

1 garlic clove, baked
(page 166) and
peeled

¼ cup extra virgin olive
oil

Juice from 1 lemon

Sea salt and freshly
ground black pepper

Puree the pepper in a blender or food processor with the garlic and olive oil. Mix in the lemon juice. Season to taste with salt and pepper.

Store in an airtight container in the refrigerator for up to 2 weeks.   MAKES ¾ CUP

secret sauce

PROTEIN, HEALTHY FATS, VEGETABLES

DETOX, LEVEL 1, LEVEL 2

½ cup tomato paste

1 tablespoon All Natural
SomerSweet

½ cup mayonnaise

1 tablespoon plus
1 teaspoon dill pickle
relish (see Note)

Sea salt and freshly
ground black pepper

Combine the tomato paste, All Natural SomerSweet, mayonnaise, and relish in a mixing bowl. Season lightly with salt and pepper.

Store in an airtight container in the refrigerator for up to 1 week.

MAKES 1 CUP

NOTE   Be sure to look for dill pickle relish, not sweet pickle relish, which can contain added sugar.

tartar sauce

HEALTHY FATS, VEGETABLES

DETOX, LEVEL 1, LEVEL 2

Place all the ingredients in a mixing bowl and season with salt and pepper. Stir until well blended.

Store in an airtight container in the refrigerator for up to 1 week. MAKES 1 1/2 CUPS

1 cup mayonnaise

1/3 cup dill pickle relish (see Note, page 152)

1/4 teaspoon Worcestershire sauce (see Note, page 45)

1 tablespoon finely chopped onion

2 teaspoons All Natural SomerSweet

2 teaspoons chopped fresh dill (optional)

2 tablespoons fresh lemon juice

Sea salt and freshly ground black pepper

chipotle and tomato salsa

HEALTHY FATS, VEGETABLES

DETOX, LEVEL 1, LEVEL 2

In a medium bowl, gently combine all the ingredients and season with salt and pepper. Serve immediately or store in an airtight container in the refrigerator for up to 3 days. MAKES 2 CUPS

2 ripe red or yellow tomatoes, medium diced

2 teaspoons adobo sauce (from canned chipotles)

1/2 red onion, finely diced

1/2 chipotle chile, finely diced

2 tablespoons extra virgin olive oil

Juice from 1/2 lime

1 tablespoon chopped fresh cilantro, or 1 1/2 teaspoons dried

Sea salt and freshly ground black pepper

vegetables
living nutrition

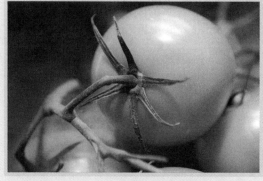

Of everything I do for my health, perhaps nothing is more important than the amount of fresh organic vegetables I give my body each day. I believe this is nature's best preventive medicine, and it happens also to be the food I love most. The thrill of my organic garden lasts all year, bringing gifts throughout the seasons. Whether you are growing your own, shopping at a farmers' market, or buying them in your local grocery store, enjoy the freshest vegetables you can find year-round; and always buy organic, if you can.

I am giddy when I see the bright yellow blossoms sprout on my zucchini plants and know the bounty is soon to follow. Once they form, I like to chop the zucchini raw, shred it into noodles, char it on the grill, or enjoy them braised or sautéed. Zucchini have a long season, so you can get creative. I feel joyous when the spiny artichokes start popping up on my plants. Every day another twenty or so are ready, so I can clip them at will. You'll discover recipes here to steam, grill, and even deep-fry them. I know they can seem expensive in stores, but knowing firsthand the amount of time it takes to grow an artichoke, I can appreciate the cost of this incredible gift from nature.

I eat tomatoes daily, especially in the summer when heirlooms are in season. Loaded with lycopene, they are heart healthy and a cancer preventative. Once you eat a home-grown tomato, it's very difficult to go back to store-bought. Most in-store tomatoes are picked green and ripened artificially. No wonder they are pink and mealy, and no wonder I wouldn't eat them as a kid! Remember, never store tomatoes in the fridge. It absolutely destroys the flavor. In the off season, I use Romas to make my signature Candied Tomatoes (page 174); I roast them in the oven with thyme, then store them in oil. They become sweet and caramelized. These tomatoes are used in many ways throughout the book—on top of fish, in making tarts, tossed into salads, or served with chicken. You'll love them.

The lesser celebrated vegetable, celery root, is also worthy of a mention. A low-glycemic alternative to insulin-spiking potatoes, Celery Root Puree (pages 161 and 162) has a delicate, creamy, subtle flavor and mashes just like potatoes. An especially important tip for those following the Sexy Forever Weight Loss Plan.

Broccoli, Brussels sprouts, green beans, peppers—this seasonal show will light up your taste buds and fill your body with immune-building nutrition. Our mothers were right when they told us, "Eat your vegetables!"

steamed artichokes with lemon-dill mayonnaise

PROTEIN, HEALTHY FATS, VEGETABLES

DETOX, LEVEL 1, LEVEL 2

Juice from 2 lemons

4 large artichokes

1 teaspoon celery seed

1 teaspoon dried dill
    weed

1 recipe Lemon-
    Dill Mayonnaise
    (page 148)

Place the lemon juice in a large bowl of water. Trim the artichokes by cutting off the stalks and removing the tough outer leaves. Slice about half of the artichoke off the top, cutting off inedible, prickly leaf tips and barely exposing the purple center or choke. Trim the tips off any remaining prickly leaves with scissors. Reserve the prepared artichokes in the bowl of lemon water to prevent discoloration.

Add about 4 inches of water, the celery seed, and dill in the bottom of a steamer. Place the artichokes in the steamer basket and steam until tender. Cooking time will vary depending on the size of the artichoke, from 40 to 60 minutes. Place each on a serving plate with a generous dollop of lemon-dill mayonnaise.   SERVES 4

tuscan deep-fried artichokes

HEALTHY FATS, VEGETABLES

DETOX, LEVEL 1, LEVEL 2

4 large artichokes

Sea salt and freshly ground black pepper

2 quarts (or more) grapeseed oil, for frying

Clean the artichokes by trimming off the bottom stalks and removing the tough outer leaves. Pull the leaves apart to slightly expose the center. Sprinkle the inside and between the leaves as best you can with salt and pepper.

Heat the oil in a deep pot until it reaches 350°F. (A candy thermometer is helpful.) The key is to have the oil at the right temperature so that the artichokes cook on the inside without burning on the outside.

Carefully add the artichokes to the hot oil and cook for approximately 10 minutes, or until crisp and golden. (You may need to cook them in batches, depending on the size of your pot.) Turn them often, pressing them against the bottom of the pan with a utensil to open the leaves. When cooked, drain on paper towels. Sprinkle again with salt and pepper and serve immediately. SERVES 4

bruschetta artichokes

HEALTHY FATS, VEGETABLES

DETOX, LEVEL 1, LEVEL 2

Juice of 1 lemon

4 large artichokes

3 ripe tomatoes, chopped

1 bunch fresh basil, chopped

¼ cup extra virgin olive oil

Sea salt and freshly ground black pepper

Place the lemon juice in a large bowl of water. Trim the artichokes by cutting off the tops of the inedible, prickly outer leaves and barely exposing the purple center of the choke. Trim the tips from the remaining leaves using scissors. Place each prepared artichoke in the bowl of lemon water to prevent discoloration.

Fill the bottom of a steamer with 4 inches of water. Place the artichokes in the steamer basket and steam until tender, 40 to 60 minutes. (Cooking time will vary depending on the size of the artichoke.) When cool, scoop out the hairy chokes, being careful to keep the heart intact.

In a separate bowl, combine the tomatoes, basil, olive oil, salt, and pepper and toss. Spoon the tomato mixture into the center of the artichokes and serve. SERVES 4

asparagus with butter and parmesan

HEALTHY FATS, VEGETABLES

DETOX, LEVEL 1, LEVEL 2

Prepare an ice bath with water and ice in a large bowl and set aside. Bring a large pot of water to a boil and add the salt. Add the asparagus and cook until tender but still a little crunchy, about 4 minutes. Remove the asparagus and immediately plunge into the ice bath to stop the cooking process. Drain the asparagus as soon as they are cool. Don't let them sit in the water too long or they will get mushy.

Heat a large skillet over medium heat and add the butter and oil. When hot, add the asparagus. Sauté just until heated through, 2 to 3 minutes. Transfer the asparagus to a platter, sprinkle with salt, pepper, and cheese, and serve immediately. SERVES 4

2 tablespoons sea salt

1 pound asparagus, washed and tough lower stems removed

2 tablespoons (1/4 stick) unsalted butter

1 tablespoon extra virgin olive oil

Sea salt and freshly ground black pepper

1/2 cup freshly grated Parmesan cheese

grilled asparagus

1 pound medium-thick
   asparagus

Extra virgin olive oil

Sea salt and freshly
   ground black pepper

Zest and juice from
   ½ lemon

HEALTHY FATS, VEGETABLES

DETOX, LEVEL 1, LEVEL 2

Heat the grill to medium.

    Wash and trim the tough ends of the asparagus. Drizzle with olive oil, then season with salt, pepper, and lemon zest.

    Place the asparagus on the grill, turning frequently for about 3 minutes. Remove from the heat and sprinkle with fresh lemon juice just before serving. SERVES 4

chilled asparagus with lemon-thyme aïoli

1 pound medium-thick
   asparagus

Extra virgin olive oil

Sea salt and freshly
   ground black pepper

1½ cups Lemon-Thyme
   Aïoli (page 245)

PROTEIN, HEALTHY FATS, VEGETABLES

DETOX, LEVEL 1, LEVEL 2

Bring a large pot of salted water to a boil. Prepare an ice bath with water and ice in a large mixing bowl.

    Trim the tough ends from the asparagus. Place into boiling water for about 4 minutes (cooking time will vary depending upon the thickness of the asparagus). Check for doneness. The asparagus should be just al dente.

    Strain immediately into a colander and plunge into the ice bath to halt the cooking process. Keep in the bath until just cooled through and remove to avoid the asparagus getting soggy. Dry on a kitchen towel and chill.

    Arrange on a platter and drizzle with olive oil, then season with salt and pepper. Serve with the aïoli. SERVES 4

cauliflower "tater" tots

PROTEIN, HEALTHY FATS, VEGETABLES

DETOX, LEVEL 1, LEVEL 2

Preheat the oven to 400°F. Lightly grease a large baking sheet.

Place the cauliflower in a 2-quart microwave-safe casserole. Add 2 tablespoons water, cover, and cook on high for 8 to 10 minutes, until very soft. Drain the cauliflower and place in the work bowl of a food processor. Add the butter, egg yolks, and Parmesan cheese. Process until the mixture is smooth. Season with salt and pepper.

Place the mixture in a piping bag fitted with a large plain tip. Pipe the cauliflower mixture in 1-inch lengths onto the baking sheet. Bake for 15 to 20 minutes, or until browned. SERVES 4 TO 6

One 1-pound bag frozen cauliflower florets, or 1 pound fresh

4 tablespoons (1/2 stick) unsalted butter, at room temperature

2 large egg yolks

1 cup freshly grated Parmesan cheese

Sea salt and freshly ground black pepper

creamy celery root puree

HEALTHY FATS, VEGETABLES

DETOX, LEVEL 1, LEVEL 2

Place about 5 cups of water in a large pot fitted with a steamer and a lid. Bring to a boil.

Chop off the roots and peel off the dark skin from the celery roots, being careful to remove all the brown. Cut each celery root into about 12 pieces and place the pieces in the steamer. Steam until very soft when poked with a fork, about 20 minutes.

Transfer the celery root to a food processor. Add the cream and butter and puree until smooth. (If you don't have a food processor, you can use an electric mixer.) Add additional cream or butter to achieve desired consistency. Sprinkle with salt and pepper. SERVES 6

3 celery roots

1/4 cup heavy cream (optional)

4 tablespoons (1/2 stick) unsalted butter

Sea salt and freshly ground black pepper

celery root puree with crispy fried onions

HEALTHY FATS, VEGETABLES
DETOX, LEVEL 1, LEVEL 2

CELERY ROOT PUREE

3 large celery roots

1/3 cup extra virgin olive oil

Sea salt and freshly ground black pepper

FRIED ONIONS

1 tablespoon olive oil

1 large onion, thinly sliced

For the celery root puree: Place about 5 cups water in a large pot fitted with a steamer and a lid. Bring to a boil.

Chop off the roots and peel off the dark skin from the celery roots, being careful to remove all the brown. Cut each celery root into about 12 pieces and place the pieces in the steamer. Steam until very soft when poked with a fork, about 20 minutes.

Transfer the celery root to a food processor. Add the olive oil and puree until smooth. (If you don't have a food processor, you can use an electric mixer.) Add additional olive oil to achieve the desired consistency. Sprinkle with salt and pepper.

For the onions: While the celery root is simmering, place the olive oil in a saucepan over medium-high heat. When hot, place the onion slices in the pan. Keep stirring while the onion starts to brown, cooking until the onion is brown and crispy, 7 to 10 minutes. Remove and drain on paper towels.

Serve the celery root with crispy fried onions on top.   SERVES 4 TO 6

braised red chard

PROTEIN, HEALTHY FATS, VEGETABLES
DETOX, LEVEL 1, LEVEL 2

2 tablespoons olive oil

1 yellow onion, finely diced

2 tablespoons (1/4 stick) unsalted butter

1/4 cup chicken stock or broth, preferably homemade (pages 30–32)

2 bunches red Swiss chard, coarsely chopped

Sea salt and freshly ground black pepper

Place a wok or large skillet over high heat. Add the olive oil and onion, and sauté for 2 to 3 minutes. Turn down the heat to medium and cook for another 7 minutes, or until lightly browned. Add the butter, stock, chard, salt, and pepper and braise for about 15 minutes.   SERVES 4

green beans with garlic vinaigrette

HEALTHY FATS, VEGETABLES

DETOX, LEVEL 1, LEVEL 2

1 pound fresh green beans

¼ cup Garlic Vinaigrette (page 142)

Steam the beans until tender and still slightly crunchy; don't overcook. Toss with the vinaigrette and serve. SERVES 4

chinese long beans

HEALTHY FATS, VEGETABLES

DETOX, LEVEL 1, LEVEL 2

1 pound Chinese long beans (or green beans)

4 tablespoons sesame oil

1 tablespoon grated fresh ginger

3 tablespoons soy sauce

Juice of 1 lemon

Freshly ground black pepper

Trim the ends off the long beans

Heat a large sauté pan over high heat. Add 3 tablespoons of the oil, then the beans, and sauté until tender, about 5 minutes. Remove the beans and set aside on a platter.

In the same pan, reduce the heat to low and add the last tablespoon of oil and the ginger. Sauté until golden, about 3 minutes. Add the soy sauce, lemon juice, and pepper. Pour the sauce over the beans and serve. SERVES 4 TO 6

spicy broccoli

HEALTHY FATS, VEGETABLES
DETOX, LEVEL 1, LEVEL 2

¼ cup grapeseed oil

2 teaspoons toasted sesame oil

6 garlic cloves, minced

1 pound broccoli florets, blanched

2 teaspoons soy sauce

1 teaspoon red pepper flakes

Heat both oils in a large skillet. Add the garlic and sauté for 1 to 2 minutes or until golden brown. Add the broccoli and cook for about 5 minutes, until it is tender but still a little crunchy. Add the soy sauce and continue to cook for 1 minute. Toss to coat the broccoli. Stir in the red pepper flakes and serve. SERVES 4

broccoli rabe with garlic and hot pepper

HEALTHY FATS, VEGETABLES
DETOX, LEVEL 1, LEVEL 2

Kosher salt

1 bunch broccoli rabe

3 tablespoons extra virgin olive oil

2 garlic cloves, thinly sliced

1 teaspoon red pepper flakes

Sea salt and freshly ground black pepper

2 tablespoons fresh lemon juice

In a large saucepan, bring 2 quarts of salted water to a boil.

Wash the broccoli rabe, cut off the bottom stems, and remove any yellow leaves. Cut into 2-inch pieces. Place the broccoli rabe into the boiling water and cook until slightly tender. Drain.

Wipe out the pan and place it back on the stove over medium heat. Add the olive oil. Add the garlic and red pepper flakes. Sauté until the garlic turns light golden brown. Add the broccoli rabe and toss well. Season with salt and pepper to taste, and the lemon juice. SERVES 4

holiday brussels sprouts with lime

HEALTHY FATS, VEGETABLES

DETOX, LEVEL 1, LEVEL 2

Cut the sprouts in half and lay flat on a chopping block. Cut each half into julienned strips.

Heat a large skillet over medium-high heat. Melt the butter, then add the sprouts and sauté until tender, 6 to 10 minutes. Season to taste with lime juice, salt, and pepper.   SERVES 12 TO 14

3 pounds Brussels sprouts

$^{1}/_{2}$ cup (1 stick) unsalted butter or olive oil

Juice from 3 to 4 limes

Sea salt and freshly ground black pepper

grilled fennel and zucchini

HEALTHY FATS, VEGETABLES

DETOX, LEVEL 1, LEVEL 2

Heat the grill to high.

Slice the zucchini very thin lengthwise. Slice the onion into thick rings, then separate. Slice the fennel into thick slices. Drizzle the vegetables with olive oil, then season with salt and pepper. Grill the zucchini for about 1 minute per side. The fennel and onion will take slightly longer. Serve immediately.   SERVES 2

2 zucchini, about 1$^{1}/_{2}$ inches in diameter

1 red onion

2 fennel bulbs, trimmed

Extra virgin olive oil

Sea salt and freshly ground black pepper

caramelized fennel

HEALTHY FATS, VEGETABLES

DETOX, LEVEL 1, LEVEL 2

4 large fennel bulbs, trimmed and thinly sliced

2 tablespoons extra virgin olive oil

2 tablespoons (^{1}/4 stick) unsalted butter

Sea salt and freshly ground black pepper

Place the fennel in a large bowl and toss with the olive oil. Heat a large skillet over medium-high heat and melt the butter. Add the fennel and reduce the heat to low. Continue cooking for about 1 hour, stirring occasionally. The fennel will become soft and caramelized to a golden brown. Season with salt and pepper. SERVES 4

baked garlic

HEALTHY FATS, VEGETABLES

DETOX, LEVEL 1, LEVEL 2

1 head garlic per serving

Extra virgin olive oil

Fresh or dried thyme

Preheat the oven to 350°F. Slice the tops off the garlic heads, exposing the cluster of cloves. Sprinkle with oil and thyme. Place in a shallow baking pan and bake for 45 minutes, or until golden brown and bubbly.

black kale

HEALTHY FATS, VEGETABLES

DETOX, LEVEL 1, LEVEL 2

2 tablespoons extra virgin olive oil

2 garlic cloves, finely minced

1 bunch black kale, cleaned very well

Juice from ^{1}/2 lemon

Sea salt and freshly ground black pepper

In a large sauté pan over medium heat, add the olive oil and garlic. Cook until the garlic is golden brown, about 1 minute. Add the kale and cook until soft, about 5 minutes. Sprinkle with the lemon juice and season with salt and pepper. Serve immediately. SERVES 2

baked caramelized onions

HEALTHY FATS, VEGETABLES

DETOX, LEVEL 1, LEVEL 2

Preheat the oven to 350°F.

Remove the skins from the onions. Trim a small amount off the base of each onion so it sits upright without tipping over. Place the onions on a cutting board and cut a deep cross on the top of each onion by slicing down from the top about halfway down the height of the onion. With an apple corer or the head of a potato peeler, carve out a small piece of the center of each onion, again starting from the top. Create a cavity large enough to fill with the garlic cloves and butter. Be careful not to carve all the way through to the bottom of the onion or the butter will run out.

Cut each garlic clove into 4 slivers, creating 16 slivers. Place 2 slivers of garlic into the cavity of each onion.

In a small dish, combine the butter and thyme. Add 1 tablespoon into the cavity of each onion. Place the onions in a roasting pan and season with salt and pepper. Drizzle half of the balsamic vinegar and half of the red wine over the onions.

Bake for 1 hour, or until the onions are soft. Then reduce the oven temperature to 300°F. Continue to cook for 1 hour more, basting frequently with the pan juices. When the juices start drying up, add the remaining balsamic vinegar and red wine. The onions are ready when they look slightly crispy and caramelized on the outside edges and are soft on the inside. The pan juices will be thick and caramelized.

To serve, spoon the thick sauce over each onion.   SERVES 8

8 onions (red, Maui, or Vidalia)

4 garlic cloves

8 tablespoons (1 stick) unsalted butter, softened

1 bunch fresh thyme, stems removed

Sea salt and freshly ground black pepper

1¹/₂ cups balsamic vinegar

1¹/₂ cups dry red wine (omit for Detox)

stuffed onions

PROTEIN, HEALTHY FATS, VEGETABLES

DETOX, LEVEL 1, LEVEL 2

6 large yellow or sweet (Vidalia or Maui) onions

Sea salt and freshly ground black pepper

2 cups Mushroom Sausage Stuffing (page 227)

1 cup chicken broth, preferably homemade (page 32)

2 tablespoons freshly grated Parmesan cheese

1 teaspoon fresh thyme leaves, or 1 teaspoon dried

1 tablespoon chopped fresh tarragon, or 1 teaspoon dried

Extra virgin olive oil, for drizzling

Preheat the oven to 350°F.

Peel each onion, then cut off the top quarter and scoop out the center until hollow. (Reserve the insides to sauté for stuffing or other use.) Season the onions inside and out with salt and pepper. Fill with the stuffing and place in a shallow baking dish. Pour the chicken broth around the onions. Sprinkle the Parmesan cheese, thyme, and tarragon on the onions and drizzle a little olive oil on top. Bake for 30 minutes, or until tender and broth has reduced by half. Spoon the reduced broth over the onions and serve.   SERVES 6

fast and easy onion rings

PROTEIN, HEALTHY FATS, VEGETABLES

LEVEL 1, LEVEL 2

4 large onions

Grapeseed or coconut oil, for deep-frying

5 large eggs

Sea salt

Peel the onions. Cut onions into ½-inch-thick slices horizontally. Separate slices into rings. Using paper towels, pat onion rings dry. This helps the egg to stick.

Heat oil to 375°F in a deep fryer or a large, deep pot.

Place the eggs in a large bowl. Beat the eggs with a fork until blended. Dip the onion rings in the egg mixture. Drop the onion rings into the hot oil. Cook for about 2 minutes, or until golden brown. Blot on paper towels. Sprinkle liberally with salt.   SERVES 4

garlic sugar snap peas

HEALTHY FATS, VEGETABLES

DETOX, LEVEL 1, LEVEL 2

Wash and trim the snap peas. Place a sauté pan on medium-high heat. When hot, add the oil and the garlic, and sauté for 1 minute. Add the snap peas and sauté until bright green and tender, about 3 minutes. Squeeze the lemon juice over the snap peas, then season with salt and white pepper to taste. Serve immediately. SERVES 4

1 pound sugar snap peas

3 tablespoons olive oil

5 garlic cloves, minced

Juice of 1/2 lemon

Sea salt and white pepper

gingered snap peas

HEALTHY FATS, VEGETABLES

DETOX, LEVEL 1, LEVEL 2

Heat the oils in a large sauté pan. Add the ginger and garlic. Cook for about 3 minutes, until both are golden brown. Add the snap peas and sauté, stirring constantly, for 1 minute. Add the soy sauce and continue cooking for 1 additional minute. Add the cayenne, stir, and transfer to a bowl. Toss the peas and let stand, loosely covered, for 5 minutes. Season with pepper and serve. SERVES 4

1/4 cup olive oil

1 tablespoon sesame oil

3 tablespoons finely chopped fresh ginger

3 garlic cloves, minced

1 pound sugar snap peas

2 tablespoons soy sauce

1/4 teaspoon cayenne

Freshly ground black pepper

smashed tuscan potatoes

8 Yukon Gold or small
 red potatoes

Sea salt

3 sprigs fresh rosemary,
 or 3 teaspoons dried

¼ cup olive oil

3 garlic cloves

1 dried red chile (chile
 de arbol)

Freshly ground black
 pepper

Place the potatoes into a medium saucepan and cover with cold water by 1 inch. Add about 2 teaspoons salt and 1 sprig of the rosemary (or 1 teaspoon of the dried). Place over high heat just until it comes to a boil, then simmer for about 20 minutes. The potatoes are done when pierced easily with a fork.

Drain the water, then set the potatoes aside to cool. When cool enough to touch, smash each with the heel of your hand.

Place a large sauté pan on medium-high heat. Add the olive oil and the whole garlic cloves. Let the garlic get crusty on one side, then turn to cook the other side. Add half the potatoes at a time (this keeps the temperature of the oil hot so the potatoes don't stick). Shake the pan to loosen the potatoes. Cook for about 2 minutes, then add the remaining potatoes, the remaining 2 sprigs of fresh rosemary (or 2 teaspoons dried), and the dried chile. Once the potatoes get crusty on one side, about 4 minutes, turn them with a spatula and cook the other side. Season with salt and pepper and serve immediately.

SERVES 2 TO 3

sinful scalloped potatoes

PROTEIN, HEALTHY FATS, INSULIN TRIGGERS

LEVEL 2

Preheat the oven to 400°F.

In a medium mixing bowl, combine all the ingredients except the potatoes and fontina cheese. Season to taste with salt and pepper.

Ladle one fourth of the cream mixture into the bottom of a Pyrex or other heavy baking dish. (The baking dish can be 9 × 9-inch or 9 × 13-inch, depending on how thick you want the finished dish.) Place the potato slices overlapping one another by one-fourth. After finishing each layer, sprinkle with salt and pepper. When finished layering all the potatoes, pour the remaining cream mixture over the top. Sprinkle with the fontina cheese and cover the dish with foil. Bake for 1 hour. Lift the foil and press the potatoes with a spatula to make sure they are evenly covered. Return to the oven until cooked completely through, about another 15 minutes. Remove the foil and cook until the potatoes are golden brown, about 15 more minutes. Serve immediately. SERVES 6

1 cup sour cream

1/2 cup mascarpone cheese or cream cheese

2 1/2 cups heavy cream

1/2 cup chicken stock or broth, preferably homemade (pages 30–32)

1/2 tablespoon chopped fresh thyme leaves

Sea salt and freshly ground black pepper

5 medium Yukon Gold potatoes, thinly sliced in rounds on a mandoline

1/4 cup freshly grated fontina cheese

grilled radicchio

2 heads radicchio

¹⁄₄ cup olive oil

2 tablespoons balsamic vinegar

Sea salt and freshly ground black pepper

HEALTHY FATS, VEGETABLES

DETOX, LEVEL 1, LEVEL 2

Heat the grill to medium high.

Slice the radicchio in half lengthwise. Rinse and pat it dry. Combine the olive oil, balsamic vinegar, and salt and pepper in a bowl. Rub the oil mixture over the halved radicchio pieces.

Place the pieces on a hot grill and cook for 3 to 5 minutes on each side. The radicchio is done when warmed with a few char marks but still has a little crunch. Serve immediately.   SERVES 4

sautéed spinach with garlic, lemon, and oil

2 tablespoons sea salt

2 pounds fresh spinach, rinsed and large stems removed

2 tablespoons olive oil

4 garlic cloves, thinly sliced

Freshly ground black pepper

Juice from 1 lemon

HEALTHY FATS, VEGETABLES

DETOX, LEVEL 1, LEVEL 2

Bring a large pot of water to a boil over high heat. Add the salt and the spinach, stirring until the spinach is just wilted, about 2 minutes. Drain the spinach and rinse thoroughly with cold water. Drain well, pressing as much liquid out of the spinach as possible.

Transfer the spinach to a chopping block and coarsely chop. Heat a large skillet over medium heat, then add the olive oil and garlic. Sauté the garlic for 1 to 2 minutes, until golden. Add the spinach and gently toss with the garlic until heated through, 2 to 3 minutes more. Season with salt, pepper, and the lemon juice. Serve immediately.   SERVES 4

spaghetti squash

HEALTHY FATS, VEGETABLES

DETOX, LEVEL 1, LEVEL 2

1 medium spaghetti squash

3 tablespoons unsalted butter

Sea salt and freshly ground black pepper

Preheat the oven to 350°F.

Slice the squash in half lengthwise. Place the halves on an oiled baking sheet, cut side down. Bake for 40 to 60 minutes or until a fork easily pierces the flesh. When cooked, scoop out the flesh into a bowl and discard the skin. Separate the flesh into strands. Toss with the butter, salt, and pepper to taste. SERVES 4

summer squash medley

HEALTHY FATS, VEGETABLES

DETOX, LEVEL 1, LEVEL 2

2 medium zucchini

2 medium crookneck squash

2 pattypan squash

2 tablespoons olive oil

1 teaspoon dried dill weed

Sea salt and freshly ground black pepper

Juice from 1 lemon

Slice the zucchini in half lengthwise and then chop crosswise, creating half-moon slices. Repeat with the crookneck squash. Quarter the pattypan squash and cut the quarters into half-moon slices as well.

Heat a wok or skillet over high heat. Add the olive oil and squash. Sprinkle with the dill, salt and pepper, and lemon juice. Sauté for 5 to 8 minutes, or until tender. SERVES 4 TO 6

squashed pattypan squash

HEALTHY FATS, VEGETABLES

DETOX, LEVEL 1, LEVEL 2

6 pattypan squash,
  quartered

3 garlic cloves,
  smashed

1 tablespoon olive oil

1 tablespoon unsalted
  butter

Sea salt and freshly
  ground black pepper

In a small saucepan, combine the squash, garlic, and olive oil. Add ½ cup water and cover. Bring to a boil, then reduce the heat and simmer for 5 to 7 minutes.

Remove from the heat and drain off the water. Remove the garlic and add the butter. Smash with a fork until chunky. Season to taste with salt and pepper. SERVES 4

candied tomatoes

HEALTHY FATS, VEGETABLES

DETOX, LEVEL 1, LEVEL 2

6 ripe large tomatoes

¼ cup olive oil

Sea salt

Preheat the oven to 325°F.

Slice the tomatoes in half crosswise. Place the tomatoes on a baking sheet, cut side up. Pour the oil over the tomatoes. Sprinkle with salt. Bake for about 2 hours, until tomatoes are wrinkled on the outside but still somewhat moist in the center. Serve warm or cool. Store in an airtight container in the refrigerator for up to 1 week. SERVES 6

stuffed tomatoes

PROTEIN, HEALTHY FATS, VEGETABLES

DETOX, LEVEL 1, LEVEL 2

Preheat the oven to 350°F.

Slice off the top of each tomato and hollow out the insides with a small spoon. Set aside.

Heat a large saucepan over medium heat. Add the olive oil and onions. Sauté the onions until browned and caramelized, about 10 minutes. Add the garlic and sauté for 1 minute longer. Add the mushrooms and sauté until browned. Add the ground meat, ½ teaspoon of the thyme, the tarragon, and the parsley. Cook 5 to 10 minutes longer, or until the chicken is lightly browned. Then add the chicken stock and cook an additional 5 minutes.

Remove the stuffing from the heat and place in a mixing bowl. Add the eggs and mix thoroughly with your hands.

Rub the inside of a shallow baking dish with olive oil. Fill the tomatoes with equal parts of the stuffing. Top each tomato with Parmesan cheese, the rest of the thyme, a sprinkling of salt and pepper, and a drizzle of olive oil. Bake for 35 minutes or until the tomatoes are soft to the touch, basting occasionally with the pan juices. (If the juices evaporate too quickly, add a little water to the bottom of the pan.)

Spoon the pan juices over the stuffed tomatoes and serve immediately. SERVES 6

12 firm, ripe medium tomatoes

4 tablespoons olive oil, plus more for drizzling

3 medium onions, thinly sliced

6 garlic cloves, finely chopped

8 ounces shiitake mushrooms, chopped

1 pound ground chicken or turkey

1 teaspoon fresh thyme leaves

1 tablespoon chopped fresh tarragon leaves

1 bunch flat-leaf parsley, chopped

½ cup chicken stock or broth, preferably homemade (pages 30–32)

2 large eggs, beaten

2 tablespoons freshly grated Parmesan cheese

Sea salt and freshly ground black pepper

broiled tomatoes

PROTEIN, HEALTHY FATS, VEGETABLES

DETOX, LEVEL 1, LEVEL 2

2 ripe tomatoes

2 tablespoons olive oil

Sea salt and freshly
  ground black pepper

¹/₄ cup freshly grated
  Parmesan cheese

1 teaspoon dried thyme

Slice the tomatoes in half crosswise. Place the tomatoes on a baking sheet, cut side up. Pour oil over the tomatoes. Sprinkle with salt, pepper, Parmesan cheese, and thyme. Broil for 5 minutes, or until the topping gets golden brown and bubbly. Serve immediately. SERVES 4

stuffed zucchini

PROTEIN, HEALTHY FATS, VEGETABLES

DETOX, LEVEL 1, LEVEL 2

6 medium zucchini,
  about 2 inches in
  diameter

2 tablespoons olive oil

1 medium onion,
  chopped

1 red bell pepper,
  cored, seeded, and
  chopped

3 garlic cloves, minced

Sea salt and freshly
  ground black pepper

Pinch of red pepper
  flakes (optional)

1 teaspoon dried
  oregano

2 large eggs

1 tablespoon freshly
  grated Parmesan
  cheese

1 teaspoon chopped
  fresh thyme leaves

Preheat the oven to 350°F.

Bring a large pot of salted water to a boil. Parboil the zucchini for 5 minutes, then remove from the water and let cool. Slice the zucchini in half lengthwise and scoop out the insides, creating a cavity to hold the stuffing. Reserve the zucchini insides in a medium bowl.

Heat a medium sauté pan over high heat. Add the olive oil, onion, and red pepper. Sauté until the onion is transparent and the pepper is soft and slightly browned, about 5 minutes. Add the garlic and sauté 1 minute longer. Remove from the heat and add to the reserved zucchini. Season with salt, pepper, red pepper flakes, if using, and oregano. Beat the eggs and stir them into the mixture, mashing the zucchini well.

Fill the zucchini shells with equal parts of the stuffing. Sprinkle with Parmesan cheese, black pepper, and thyme. Place in an ungreased shallow baking dish and bake for 35 minutes, until the stuffing is golden brown and bubbly. Serve 2 per person. SERVES 6

zucchini noodles

HEALTHY FATS, VEGETABLES

DETOX, LEVEL 1, LEVEL 2

12 zucchini, about
1 1/2 inches in
diameter

2 tablespoons olive oil

Sea salt and freshly
ground black pepper

With a good potato peeler, create zucchini "noodles" by starting at the top of the zucchini and peeling wide ribbons down the length of each. Continue making ribbons as you turn the zucchini to get all the green part off first. When the center portion becomes too thin, set it aside and start a new zucchini. (Use the leftover centers in soups or salads.)

Heat a large skillet on medium-high heat. Add the olive oil and the zucchini noodles. Sauté the noodles for 2 to 3 minutes. Season with salt and pepper. SERVES 4

SERVING SUGGESTIONS Use zucchini noodles in place of pasta. Toss them with Basil-Parsley Pesto (page 150). Or serve with Pan-Fried Garlic Lemon Shrimp (page 253) or with Caroline's Meat Sauce (page 281).

cumin-scented zucchini

HEALTHY FATS, VEGETABLES

DETOX, LEVEL 1, LEVEL 2

6 medium zucchini,
about 1 1/2 inches in
diameter

1 tablespoon ground
cumin

3 tablespoons olive oil

3 garlic cloves, minced

Sea salt and freshly
ground black pepper

Lemon wedges

Quarter the zucchini lengthwise. Cut each strip into ½-inch pieces. Each piece will be triangular in shape.

Heat a 10-inch sauté pan over medium heat. Add the cumin and stir for 10 seconds to bring out the flavor. Add the oil and heat for 30 seconds. Add the garlic, then the zucchini. Turn the heat to high and sauté for 2 minutes. Season with salt and pepper. Squeeze lemon juice over the zucchini and serve. SERVES 4

grilled vegetable towers

2 medium zucchini, sliced on the diagonal into $1/2$-inch slices

1 red onion, cut into $1/2$-inch rings

1 red bell pepper, cored, quartered, and seeded

1 yellow bell pepper, cored, quartered, and seeded

1 fennel bulb, trimmed and cut into $1/2$-inch slices

1 pint cherry tomatoes

1 large eggplant, cut into $1/2$-inch-thick slices

Olive oil

Sea salt and freshly ground black pepper

$1/2$ cup balsamic vinegar

8 ounces feta cheese, crumbled

Heat the grill to medium high.

Brush all the vegetables with a little olive oil. Season with salt and pepper. Place as many vegetables on the grill as will fit at one time. The onions, pepper, and fennel will take the longest. Grill until tender. You want them to have char marks, but not to be burned.

Place the vinegar in a small saucepan over high heat. Reduce by half or more, until thickened and syrupy.

Stack the grilled vegetables into 4 towers. Start with a slice of eggplant, then the onions, then the red pepper, the fennel, the yellow pepper, then the zucchini. (Stack another layer high, if you wish, with the leftover vegetables.) Strew the tomatoes around the plate. Crumble the feta cheese over the top. Drizzle the hot balsamic vinegar over the top and serve.   SERVES 4

caramelized root vegetables

HEALTHY FATS, VEGETABLES

DETOX, LEVEL 1, LEVEL 2

In a medium sauté pan over medium heat, add the olive oil and vegetables. Cook slowly. As the vegetables begin to caramelize, add 1 tablespoon of the butter. Continue to cook for 10 minutes. Add the remaining butter. Season to taste with salt and pepper and serve immediately.   SERVES 6

1 tablespoon olive oil

1 celery root, peeled and cut into small pieces

1 turnip, peeled and cut into small pieces

1 rutabaga, peeled and cut into small pieces

2 tablespoons (^{1}/4 stick) unsalted butter

Sea salt and freshly ground black pepper

vegetables provençal

HEALTHY FATS, VEGETABLES

DETOX, LEVEL 1, LEVEL 2

   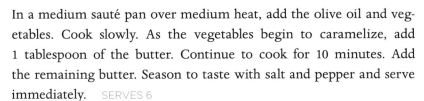

Heat the olive oil in a large skillet. Add the onions and cook over medium-low heat until browned and caramelized, about 30 minutes. Add the garlic and cook for 1 minute. Turn up the heat to medium high and add the zucchini (and additional oil if the pan seems too dry). Cook until tender, about 8 minutes.

Sprinkle with thyme leaves, salt, and pepper. Add the tomatoes and stir until combined. Continue cooking until the tomatoes are heated through, about 5 minutes more.   SERVES 6

^{1}/3 cup olive oil, plus more as needed

3 medium onions, sliced

5 garlic cloves, thinly sliced

3 medium zucchini, sliced

8 sprigs fresh thyme

Sea salt and freshly ground black pepper

12 Candied Tomatoes (page 174)

summer stir-fry

2 tablespoons olive oil

1 tablespoon sesame oil

2 yellow summer
squash, julienned

2 small zucchini,
julienned

1 leek, white part only,
julienned

1 pound asparagus, cut
into bite-size pieces

2 tablespoons soy
sauce

Juice of ½ lemon

Hot chili oil (optional)

Heat a wok over high heat. Add the olive and sesame oils and the yellow squash, stirring constantly for about 2 minutes, or until tender and still a little crunchy. Remove the squash and set aside. Add the zucchini and cook for about 2 minutes; add more oil as needed. Remove and set aside. Repeat with the leek, then the asparagus.

Place all the vegetables back in the wok with the soy sauce and lemon juice. Toss until well coated. Remove from the heat and serve immediately. Add a couple of dashes of hot chili oil as desired.   SERVES 4

stir-fried vegetables

HEALTHY FATS, VEGETABLES

DETOX, LEVEL 1, LEVEL 2

2 tablespoons grape-
seed or coconut oil

6 cups coarsely
chopped vegetables
(baby bok choy,
broccoli, snow peas,
celery, onion, yellow
or red bell peppers)

5 to 10 dashes soy
sauce

Juice from 1 lemon

1 teaspoon toasted
sesame oil

A few drops hot chili oil,
or ½ teaspoon red
pepper flakes

Place a wok or large frying pan over high heat. Add a little grapeseed or coconut oil. Add the vegetables in small batches and cook quickly to keep the wok hot. As each batch is cooked, place the vegetables on a platter until all are cooked (tender when poked with a fork, but not soggy).

Put all the vegetables back in the wok or frying pan and add the soy sauce, lemon juice, sesame oil, and hot chili oil or red pepper flakes.   SERVES 4

The inspiration for every recipe comes from nature. It tells me on a daily basis what is at its peak.

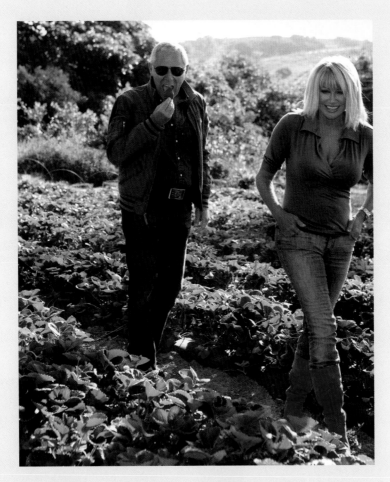

Here's a look at my local journey for the finest ingredients, as close to the source as possible.

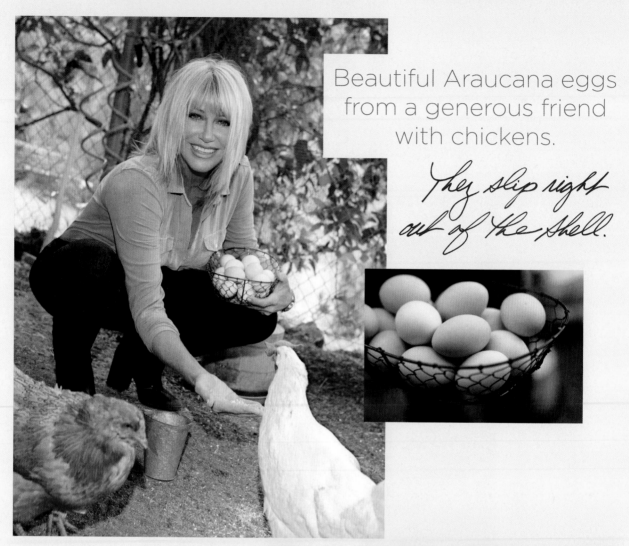

Beautiful Araucana eggs from a generous friend with chickens.

They slip right out of the shell.

We always eat whatever fruit is in season.

Tangelos bursting with flavor.

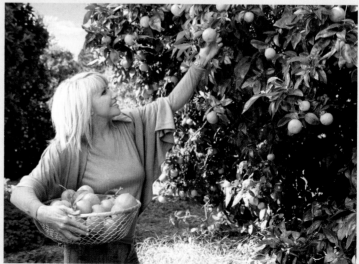

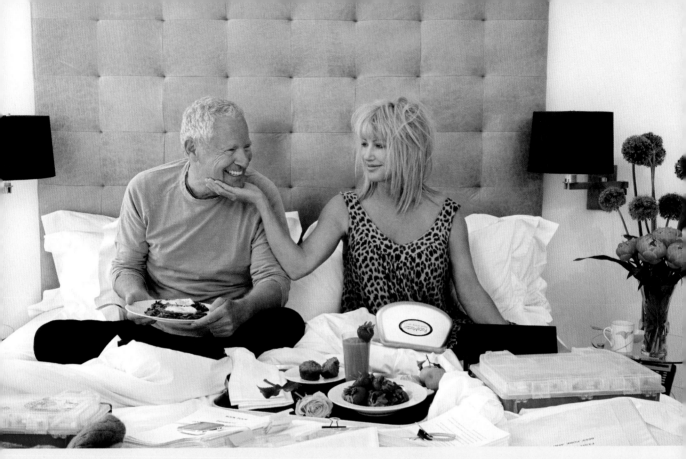

Breakfast in bed with my Al...

very sexy—along with our ipads, a Gacemaster, trunks of Vitamins, and a manuscript!

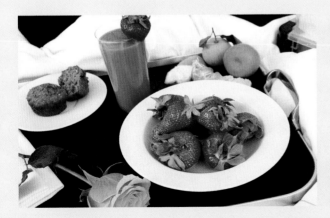

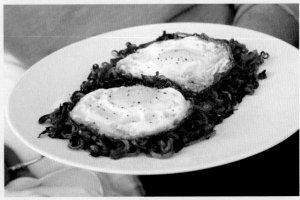

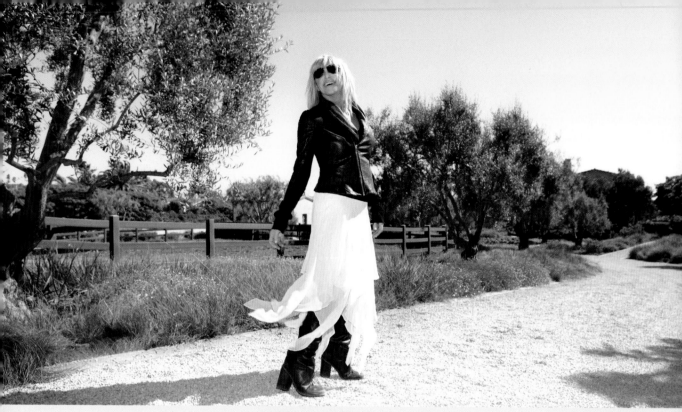

Off to Malibu Olive Company
for my staple—extra virgin olive oil

liquid gold for health, taste, and most every recipe in this book.

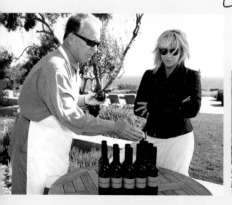
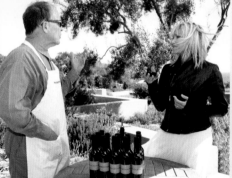
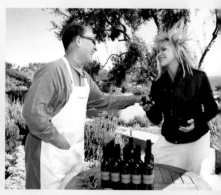

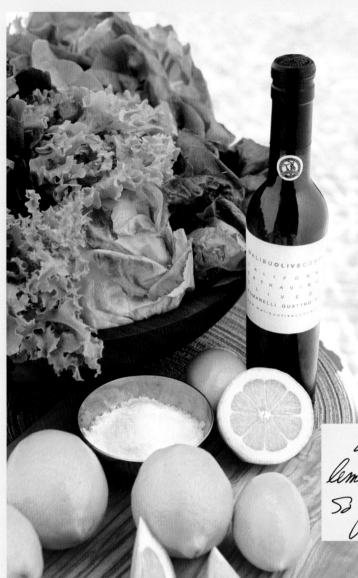

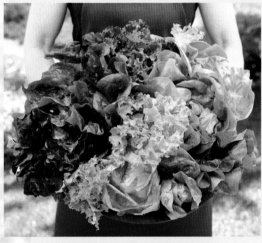

Thrilling bounty of
lettuces from my
organic garden.

*drizzle of oil, squeeze of
lemon, sprinkle of sea salt.
So fresh, it tastes alive!*

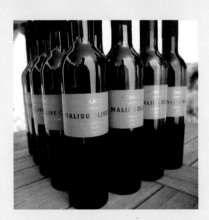

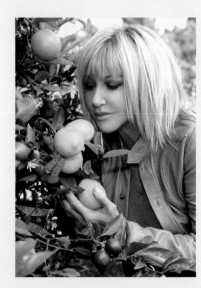

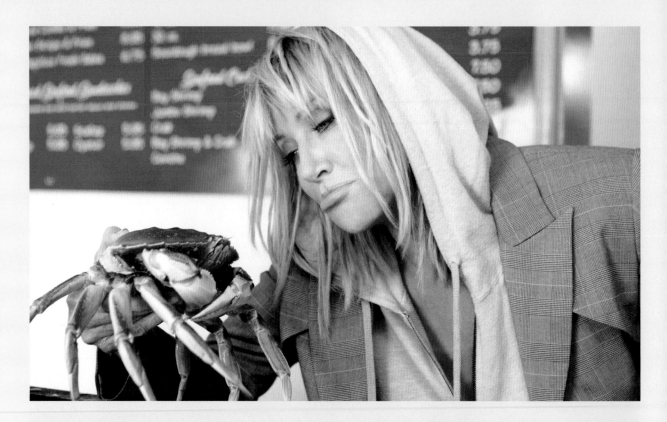

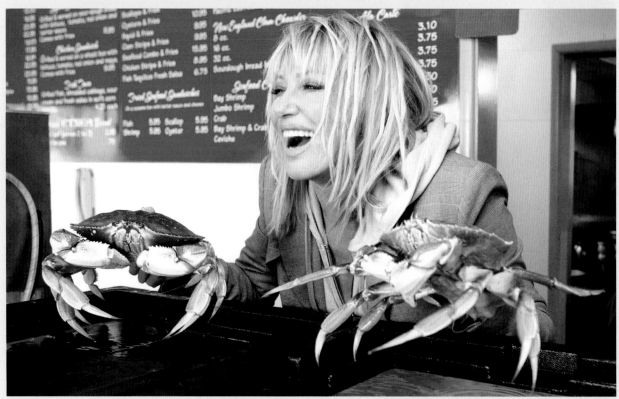

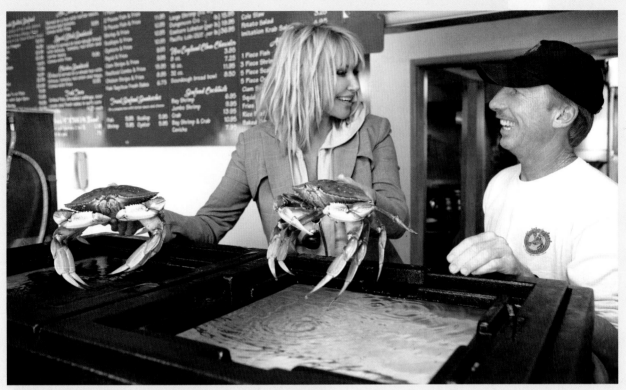

The locals know the best hangouts—Malibu Seafood.

My friend John helps me pick a couple of crabs for my delicious crab bisque.

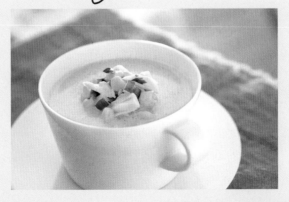

my favorite things...

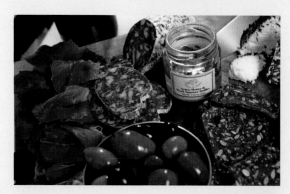

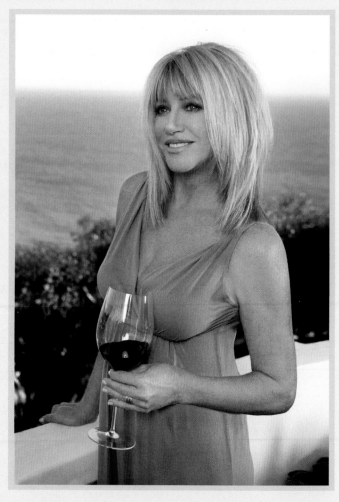

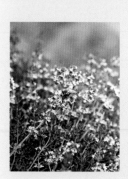

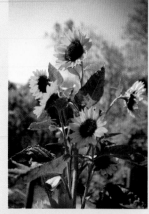

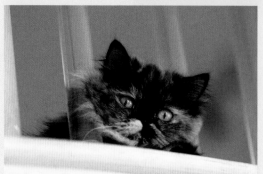

The ocean, charcuterie, herbed goat cheese, truffle honey, a glass of red, bees on blossoming thyme, happy sunflowers... and Betty.

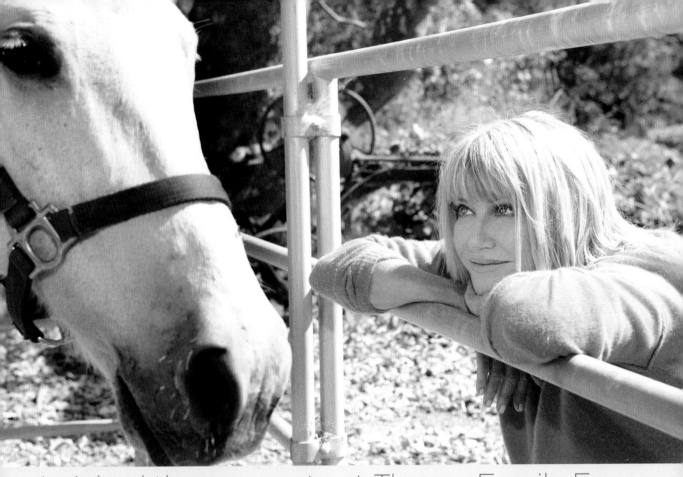

I picked these carrots at Thorne Family Farm

but ended up feeding all of them to Lulabell!

Fast Friends.

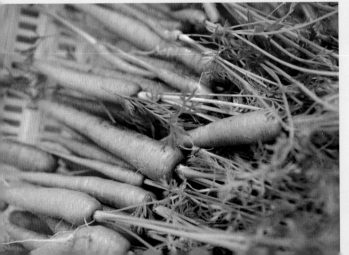

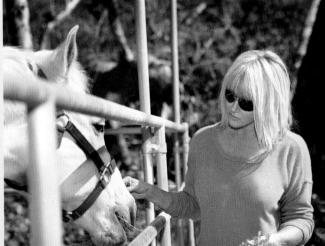

We see Larry once a week at his local organic farm.

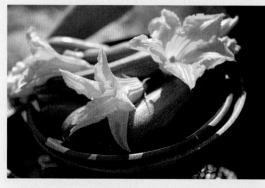

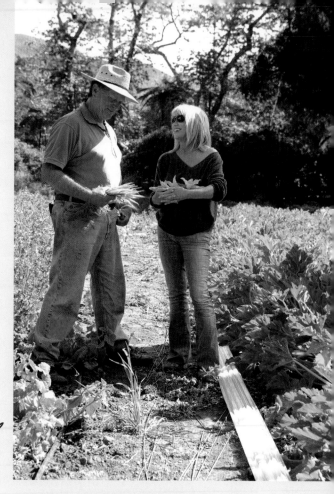

Talk about this week's "special"... Zucchini with stunning blossoms.

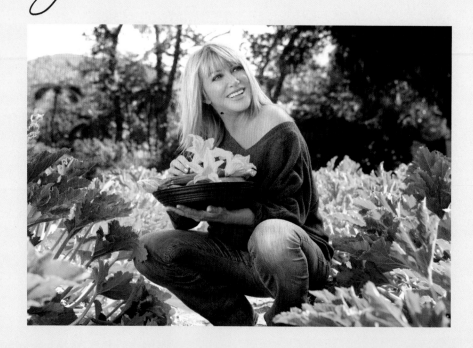

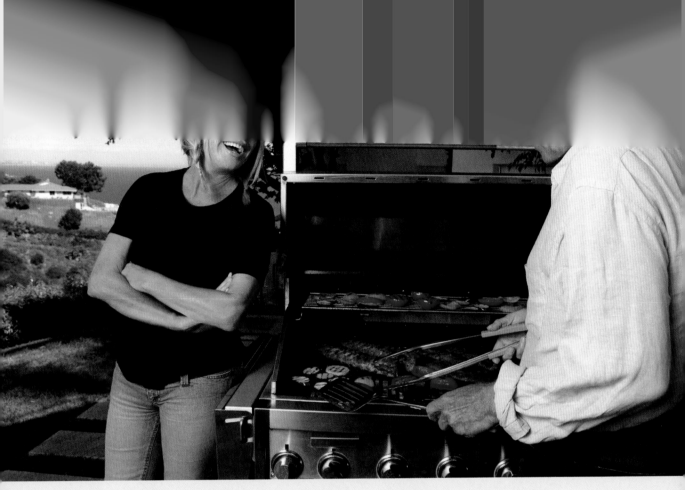

Alan mans the grill

with ribs, carne asada, and vibrant grilled vegetables.

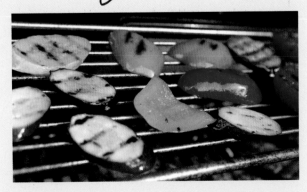

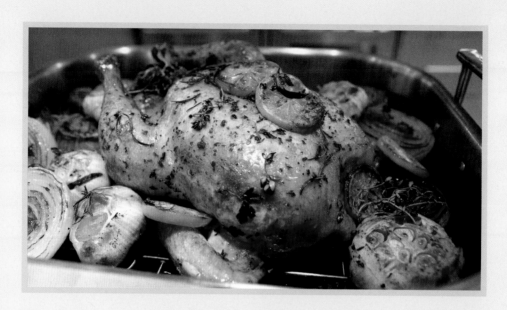

Zannie's Lemon Herb Chicken

1. Drizzle a 5 lb. chicken with olive oil.

2. Slice the top off a head of garlic and rub all over.

3. Squeeze a lemon, then toss it inside the cavity.

4. Liberally sprinkle with sea salt...

5. And freshly cracked black pepper.

6. Add oil, onions, garlic.

7. Cover with fresh tarragon, sage, rosemary, and thyme.

8. Top with lemon slices and butter.

9. Roast at 350° for two hours.

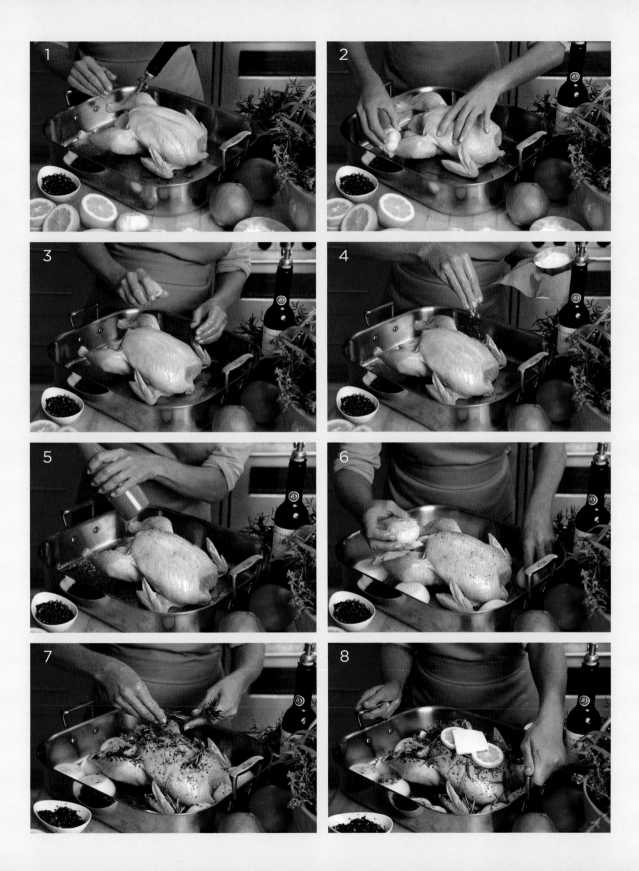

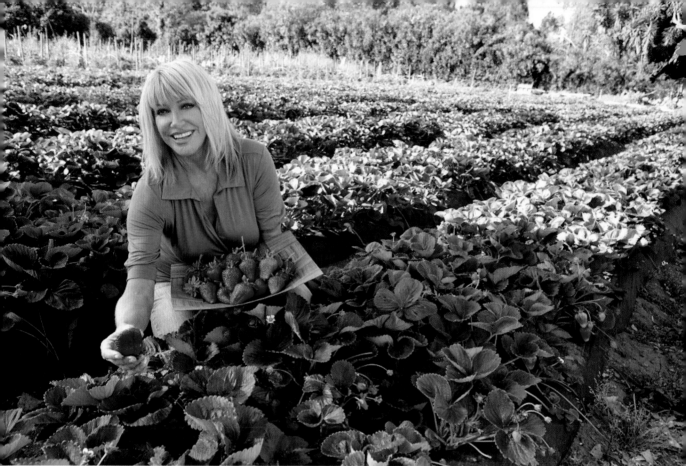

Strawberries—nothing compares to the taste fresh off the vine.

Perfect for my fruit smoothie.

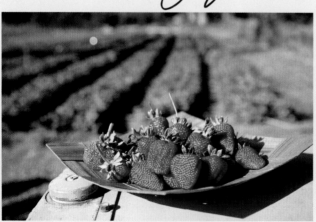

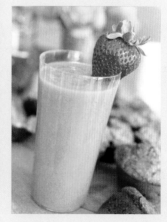

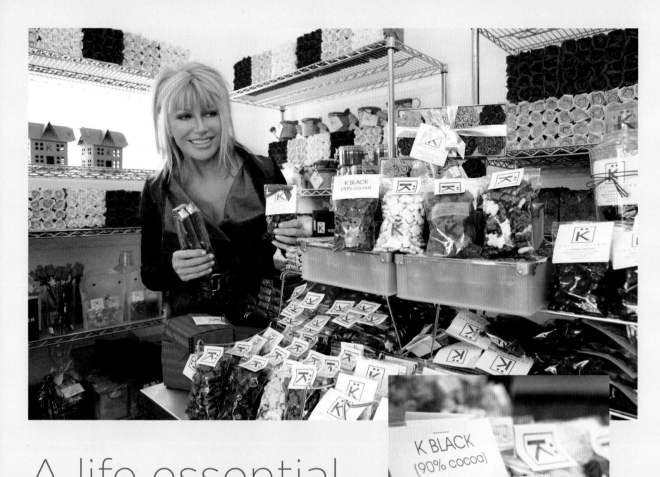

A life essential... chocolate!

K BLACK
(90% cocoa)

Decadent Chocolate Cake perfectly paired with a plump Strawberry.

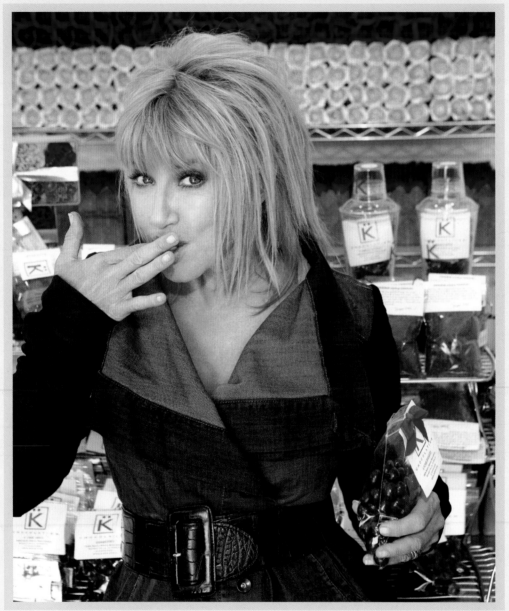

Mmmmmmmm...

to life, love, and food!
Love,
Suzanne

roasted vegetable lasagne

VEGETABLES, CARBOHYDRATES

DETOX, LEVEL 1, LEVEL 2

Preheat the oven to 425°F.

Lay the zucchini, eggplant, and tomatoes cut side up on baking sheets. Sprinkle with salt, pepper, and 1 tablespoon of thyme. Roast until golden brown. The zucchini and eggplant will take about 15 minutes, the tomatoes about 45 minutes. Lower the oven temperature to 350°F.

Combine the ricotta, garlic, remaining 2 tablespoons thyme, and salt and pepper in a bowl.

Cook the pasta according to package instructions. Rinse with cool water, and lay the pieces out flat so they don't stick together.

To assemble the lasagne, pour a thin layer of tomato sauce (½ cup) on the bottom of a 13 × 9-inch pan. Lay 3 lasagna noodles lengthwise in the pan, then add half of the ricotta and garlic mixture, a layer of roasted peppers, and a layer of zucchini, then another layer of pasta, the rest of the cheese mixture, another ½ cup of sauce, then the eggplant and tomatoes. Top with a layer of pasta, ending with more tomato sauce.

Cover with foil and bake about 45 minutes or until bubbling. Remove from the oven and let stand for 10 minutes before serving.   SERVES 6

4 medium zucchini, sliced lengthwise into $\frac{1}{8}$-inch slices

1 large eggplant, sliced lengthwise into $\frac{1}{8}$-inch slices

20 medium tomatoes, cut in half crosswise

Sea salt and freshly ground black pepper

3 tablespoons chopped fresh thyme leaves

2 cups nonfat ricotta cheese

1 head Baked Garlic (page 166)

1 pound whole-grain lasagna noodles

1 recipe Tomato Basil Sauce (page 188)

8 Roasted Red Peppers (page 134) or jarred roasted peppers in water

FOR LEVEL 1 AND LEVEL 2 For Detox, this recipe contains no added fats. For additional flavor in Level 1 and Level 2, add olive oil to the roasted vegetables, and add ¼ cup freshly grated Parmesan cheese and ½ cup grated mozzarella to the ricotta mixture.

eggplant parmesan

HEALTHY FATS, VEGETABLES
DETOX, LEVEL 1, LEVEL 2

2 firm medium
eggplants (about
2 pounds)

2 quarts grapeseed oil

Sea salt and freshly
ground black pepper

2 cups Sweet Tomato
Sauce (recipe
follows)

1 pound mozzarella
cheese, thinly sliced

1 cup freshly grated
Parmesan cheese

1/2 cup loosely packed,
roughly chopped
fresh basil leaves

Preheat the oven to 400°F.

Cut the eggplants lengthwise into very thin slices.

Heat the oil in a large skillet or deep-fryer to about 360°F. Fry 2 or 3 slices of eggplant at a time until golden brown, about 4 minutes. Drain the slices on paper towels. Season with salt and pepper.

Spoon several tablespoons of the tomato sauce into a 9 × 13-inch casserole dish. Layer half the fried eggplant over the sauce. Spoon another thin layer of sauce over the eggplant. Cover with half the mozzarella, then about half of the Parmesan cheese. Layer on the rest of the eggplant, then a little more tomato sauce, remaining mozzarella, and the other half of the Parmesan cheese. Sprinkle with the fresh basil.

Bake until the cheese is bubbling and melted, about 40 minutes. Let the casserole cool for about 10 minutes, then cut into squares and serve. SERVES 6 TO 8

sweet tomato sauce

HEALTHY FATS, VEGETABLES
DETOX, LEVEL 1, LEVEL 2

   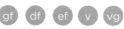

1 large onion
8 ripe tomatoes, or one 28-ounce can plum tomatoes, drained
¼ cup olive oil
3 garlic cloves, minced
Sea salt and freshly ground black pepper

Chop the onion in a food processor until finely minced. Coarsely chop the tomatoes in a food processor or blender.

Heat a medium skillet on medium heat. Add the olive oil. When the oil is hot, add the minced onion and cook until translucent, 4 to 5 minutes. Add the garlic and cook for another minute. Add the tomatoes and reduce the heat. Simmer for 45 minutes, until sauce thickens a little. Season with salt and pepper. MAKES ABOUT 2 CUPS

susie's eggplant manicotti

TOMATO SAUCE
2 pounds ripe
   tomatoes, washed
   and quartered

1 cup chopped carrots
   (omit for Detox and
   Level 1)

1 cup chopped celery

³/4 cup chopped onion

¹/4 cup heavy cream

EGGPLANT
2 large eggplants

Sea salt

Extra virgin olive oil

FILLING
1 cup nonfat ricotta
   cheese

2 tablespoons freshly
   grated Parmesan
   cheese

1 large egg yolk

Sea salt and freshly
   ground black pepper

Freshly grated nutmeg

³/4 pound fresh
   spinach, washed and
   large stems removed

1 bunch fresh basil,
   leaves cut into
   julienne

For the tomato sauce: Cook the tomatoes in a large saucepan over low heat until the juice is released, about 10 minutes. Add the carrots, celery, and onion. Simmer over low heat for about 1 hour, or until most of liquid has boiled away. Cool slightly and puree in a food processor or blender. Return to the pan over low heat and reduce by about a third. Stir in the cream and simmer 10 to 15 minutes (or freeze at this point).

For the eggplant: Peel the eggplants and slice lengthwise into ¹/8-inch-thick pieces. Place the slices in a colander and sprinkle with salt. Let sit for about 30 minutes. Rinse well, then pat the slices dry.

Preheat the oven to 350°F.

Lightly oil a cookie sheet. Place the eggplant slices in a single layer and lightly brush with oil. Bake for 20 minutes. The eggplant will become soft. Don't overcook the slices or they will become brittle and won't work for this recipe.

Reduce oven to 325°F.

For the filling: In a mixing bowl, combine the ricotta, Parmesan, egg yolk, salt and pepper, and grated nutmeg. Place the spinach in a covered steamer basket over boiling water and steam for 3 minutes. Drain well, then chop and stir into the ricotta mixture.

To assemble the manicotti: Place 1 tablespoon of filling near the edge of each slice of eggplant. Roll up and place on lightly greased cookie sheet, forming manicotti-like tubes. (These tubes can be made in advance and refrigerated overnight.)

Bake at 325°F for 20 to 30 minutes. Spoon a bit of sauce on individual serving plates and top each plate with 3 or 4 eggplant manicotti. Spoon on more sauce and garnish with basil. Serve immediately. SERVES 8

rice, beans, pasta, and grains

the whole deal

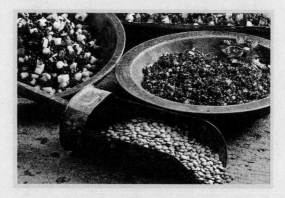

Whole-grain goodness should not be confused with poor reviled refined carbohydrates. Once we all understood the effects of white flour and sugar on our health and waistlines, we turned our backs on carbs altogether. What do they say about the baby going out with the bathwater?

Refined carbohydrates such as white flour, white rice, white pasta, and white bread spike insulin levels and are, indeed, not worthy of a spot on the Sexy Forever plan, nor in this cookbook. However, their whole-grain counterparts are delicious, nutty, earthy, and wonderfully acceptable in proper portions. (Learn more about this at SexyForever.com.) You'll discover whole new flavor sensations with recipes for Farro Risotto (page 194), Parsnip Garlic Ravioli (page 192), Sautéed Herb Quinoa (page 197), Forbidden Rice (page 195), French Lentils (page 201), and many more.

While several whole grains contain gluten, if you are allergic or intolerant, consider pasta made from brown rice (I love Tinkyada Pasta Joy) or even better from quinoa—an ancient Incan super-food that happens to be great as pasta. (I prefer Andean Farm brand.) And you won't find any gluten in Macaroni and Cheese (page 187), where the macaroni is made from eggs. I have found delicious ways to provide your favorite tastes, with a little twist on the classics.

The anti-carb revolution simply needs to be a "carbohydrate evolution," meaning we include the right carbs, in the right amounts. Eating carbs is oh so satisfying. Doing it right is oh so healthy.

macaroni and cheese

PROTEIN, HEALTHY FATS

DETOX, LEVEL 1, LEVEL 2

4 cups heavy cream

2$\frac{1}{2}$ cups shredded Cheddar cheese

Pinch of ground nutmeg

Pinch of cayenne

8 Egg Crêpes (page 35), cut into $\frac{1}{4}$-inch strips

Sea salt and freshly ground black pepper

Preheat the oven to 350°F. Butter an 8-inch square glass baking dish. Set aside.

Place the cream in a heavy medium saucepan. Bring to a boil, reduce the heat slightly, and let boil gently for 10 minutes, or until reduced by half. Lower the heat and add 1½ cups of the Cheddar cheese, the nutmeg, and cayenne. Stir until the cheese melts and sauce is smooth.

Place the crêpe strips in the prepared baking dish. Pour the sauce over and stir to coat. Top with the remaining 1 cup cheese. Bake for 20 minutes, or until the cheese is bubbly and beginning to brown. Season with salt and pepper. Serve hot. SERVES 4

quinoa linguine with candied tomatoes

HEALTHY FATS, VEGETABLES, CARBOHYDRATES

LEVEL 1, LEVEL 2

$\frac{1}{2}$ pound quinoa or whole-grain linguine

$\frac{1}{4}$ cup extra virgin olive oil

1 red onion, thinly sliced

2 garlic cloves, finely chopped

12 Candied Tomatoes (page 174)

Zest of 1 lemon

1 bunch fresh basil, leaves only

Red pepper flakes

Sea salt and freshly ground black pepper

In a large sauté pan over high heat, add 2 tablespoons of the olive oil and the onion and cook until the onion is caramelized and soft, 7 to 10 minutes. Add the garlic, tomatoes, lemon zest, and basil. Cook until the tomatoes soften, about 10 minutes.

Cook the pasta according to the package instructions. Drain the pasta and add 2 cups of the cooked linguine to the sauté pan. Toss together and add the remaining 2 tablespoons olive oil, the red pepper flakes, and salt and pepper to taste. Serve immediately. SERVES 2

penne with tomato basil sauce

Two 28-ounce cans
tomatoes, coarsely
chopped with juice

1 medium onion,
chopped

6 garlic cloves, very
thinly sliced

Sea salt and freshly
ground black pepper

20 fresh basil leaves,
stacked, rolled, and
thinly sliced

1 pound whole-grain
penne pasta

Over medium-high heat, warm about ⅓ cup of the juice from the peeled tomatoes in a large saucepan. Add the onion and sauté until soft, about 7 minutes. Then add the garlic and sauté another 3 minutes. (If the tomato juice is bubbling too much, turn the heat down to medium.) Add the remaining tomatoes and their juice. Lower the heat and simmer for 20 minutes. Add salt and pepper to taste. Stir and cook for an additional 5 minutes. Turn off the heat and add the basil.

Cook the pasta according to the package instructions. Toss with the sauce and serve immediately.   SERVES 6

FOR LEVEL 1 AND LEVEL 2 For Detox, this recipe contains no added fats. For additional flavor in Level 1 and Level 2, start the sauce by sautéing the onion for about 10 minutes (until golden brown) in about ½ cup extra virgin olive oil. Add the garlic and cook until just pale gold. Turn down the heat and add the tomatoes with their juice. Finish as above.

penne all'arrabbiata

HEALTHY FATS, VEGETABLES, CARBOHYDRATES

LEVEL 1, LEVEL 2

Place a large skillet over medium-high heat. Add the olive oil and the garlic. Sauté until golden, 2 minutes. Add the tomatoes and salt to taste and bring to a boil. Lower the heat to simmer, add the red pepper flakes, and cook for 20 to 25 minutes. The sauce will reduce and thicken.

Cook the pasta according to the package instructions. Drain in a colander, reserving ½ cup of the pasta water.

Place the penne, pasta water, and tomato sauce back into a large saucepan and toss until each piece is well coated. Add the oregano and basil. Adjust the seasonings. Serve immediately.   SERVES 4

2 tablespoons olive oil

6 garlic cloves, minced

Two 28-ounce cans crushed Italian plum tomatoes with juice

Sea salt

2 teaspoons red pepper flakes, or more if desired

1 pound brown rice, quinoa, or whole-grain penne

½ teaspoon dried oregano

10 fresh basil leaves, julienned

spinach and ricotta ravioli with candied tomato sauce

HEALTHY FATS, VEGETABLES,
CARBOHYDRATES, INSULIN TRIGGERS
LEVEL 2

RAVIOLI

15 ounces nonfat ricotta cheese

$^{1}/_{2}$ pound fresh spinach, chopped, then steamed for 3 minutes

3 shallots, finely chopped

$^{1}/_{2}$ cup freshly grated Parmesan cheese, plus additional for serving

2 teaspoons finely chopped fresh basil, or 1 teaspoon dried

1 tablespoon finely chopped flat-leaf parsley, or $^{1}/_{2}$ tablespoon dried

Sea salt and freshly ground black pepper

1 package (30) square wonton wrappers, defrosted if frozen

CANDIED TOMATO SAUCE

12 Candied Tomatoes (page 174)

2 tablespoons extra virgin olive oil

For the ravioli: Place the ricotta, spinach, shallots, Parmesan, basil, parsley, and salt and pepper in a large mixing bowl. Stir filling until well combined.

Place a single wonton wrapper on a cutting board. Have a small glass of water standing by. Place a teaspoon of filling just off the center of the wrapper. Dip your finger in the water and wet the bottom two edges of the wonton. Fold the wonton in half to form a triangle. Gently press the edges together to force out air. Repeat to form the remaining ravioli, placing in a single layer on a cookie sheet lightly floured with whole wheat flour; cover with a light kitchen towel. (You can also place them in freezer bags, separating the layers with parchment paper. They will keep in the freezer for up to 3 months.)

To make the sauce: Puree the candied tomatoes with the olive oil then heat in a saucepan until bubbling.

When ready to cook, bring a large pot of salted water to a boil. Add the ravioli, one at a time, carefully dropping them into the water. The ravioli are done shortly after they rise to the surface, or in about 5 minutes. Remove with a slotted spoon and place in individual serving bowls.

Top with a spoonful of sauce and a sprinkle of Parmesan cheese. SERVES 4

pasta with garlic and pine nuts

HEALTHY FATS, VEGETABLES, CARBOHYDRATES

LEVEL 1, LEVEL 2

Heat the olive oil in a large skillet. Add the garlic and cook until lightly browned, about 3 minutes. Add the pine nuts, then the parsley, salt, and pepper. Continue stirring until the pine nuts start to brown.

Cook the pasta according to the package instructions. Drain, reserving 3 tablespoons of the water. Add the pasta and the reserved water to the sauce and toss until heated through and completely coated. SERVES 4 TO 6

¼ cup extra virgin olive oil

6 garlic cloves, minced

½ cup pine nuts

1 bunch flat-leaf parsley, chopped

Sea salt and freshly ground black pepper

1 pound whole-grain linguine or spaghetti

whole-grain pasta primavera

HEALTHY FATS, VEGETABLES, CARBOHYDRATES

LEVEL 1, LEVEL 2

Place a large pot of salted water over high heat and bring to a boil.

Slice the zucchini, yellow squash, peppers, and snap peas into julienne strips of similar size. Heat a large skillet over medium heat. Add the olive oil and garlic and cook until golden, 1 to 2 minutes. Turn the heat to high and add the vegetables, sautéing until just tender, 4 to 5 minutes.

Add the pasta to the boiling water and cook according to the package instructions. Drain, reserving 3 tablespoons of the water. Add the pasta and the reserved water to the sautéed vegetables. Toss everything together and season liberally with salt and pepper. Add more olive oil, if necessary, to coat all the pasta. Sprinkle with the chopped parsley and Parmesan cheese. SERVES 4

Kosher salt

2 zucchini

2 yellow squash

1 red bell pepper

1 yellow bell pepper

2 pounds snap peas

3 tablespoons olive oil

4 garlic cloves, minced

1 pound whole-grain pasta

Sea salt and freshly ground black pepper

2 bunches flat-leaf parsley, chopped

Freshly grated Parmesan cheese

parsnip garlic ravioli with mushroom ragout

HEALTHY FATS, VEGETABLES,
CARBOHYDRATES, INSULIN TRIGGERS

LEVEL 2

MUSHROOM RAGOUT

2 tablespoons olive oil

2 medium onions, thinly sliced

1 tablespoon unsalted butter

1 pound portobello mushrooms, thinly sliced

³/4 pound white mushrooms, thinly sliced

3 garlic cloves, minced

1 teaspoon chopped fresh sage leaves

Sea salt and freshly ground black pepper

One 28- to 32-ounce can whole tomatoes, drained, coarsely chopped, juice reserved

RAVIOLI

1 package (30) square wonton wrappers, defrosted if frozen

Parsnip Puree with Roasted Garlic (recipe follows)

For the mushroom ragout: In a large skillet over medium heat, add the olive oil and sliced onions. Cook for 10 minutes, until the onions are browned and caramelized, about 15 minutes. Stir often. Add the butter and stir until melted. Add all of the mushrooms, the garlic, sage, and salt and pepper to taste. Sauté, stirring constantly, for about 15 minutes, or until the mushroom liquid is evaporated. Stir in the tomatoes and reserved juice. Cook uncovered for 30 minutes. Stir occasionally.

For the ravioli: Place a wonton wrapper on a work surface and mound 1 tablespoon of the parsnip puree in the center. Brush the edges of the wrapper with water and fold the wrapper in half to form a triangle. Press securely on the edges to force out air. Repeat with the remaining wrappers, placing them on a cookie sheet lightly floured with whole wheat flour; cover with a light kitchen towel. Refrigerate until ready to use.

To finish: Cook the ravioli in a large pot of boiling salted water for approximately 5 minutes, or until they rise to the surface and are tender. Do not let the water boil vigorously once the ravioli have been added.

Immediately transfer the ravioli to serving plates. Top with mushroom ragout and serve. SERVES 2

parsnip puree with roasted garlic

HEALTHY FATS, VEGETABLES, INSULIN TRIGGERS

LEVEL 2

2 garlic cloves
2 tablespoons olive oil
1 pound parsnips
4 ounces cream cheese, softened
Sea salt and freshly ground black pepper

Preheat the oven to 350°F.

Put the garlic into a small pan with the olive oil. Roast in the oven for 30 minutes or sauté on top of the stove for 15 minutes.

Wash and peel the parsnips. Cut into 1-inch pieces and put into a 2-quart saucepan with just enough water to cover them. Cover and cook until tender, approximately 15 minutes. Drain off the water and mash the parsnips with the cream cheese and roasted garlic. Season to taste with salt and pepper.   MAKES 1 CUP

soba noodles

HEALTHY FATS, CARBOHYDRATES

LEVEL 1, LEVEL 2

One 8-ounce package
soba noodles

2 teaspoons soy sauce

1 teaspoon rice wine
vinegar

1 tablespoon olive oil

1 tablespoon chopped
fresh chives

Sea salt and freshly
ground black pepper

Cook the noodles according to the package instructions. After the noodles are cooked, run them under cold water to stop them from further cooking. Place the noodles into a medium bowl. Add the soy sauce, vinegar, oil, chives, and salt and pepper to taste.   SERVES 4

farro risotto

PROTEIN, HEALTHY FATS, VEGETABLES, CARBOHYDRATES

LEVEL 1, LEVEL 2

4 cups chicken stock
or broth, preferably
homemade
(pages 30–32)

1 tablespoon extra
virgin olive oil

1/2 onion, medium diced

1 cup raw farro

2 tablespoons (1/4 stick)
unsalted butter

1/4 cup freshly grated
Parmesan cheese

Sea salt and freshly
ground black pepper

In a medium saucepan, bring the chicken broth to a boil and reduce to a simmer.

In a separate saucepan over medium heat, add the oil and onion and sauté until translucent, about 5 minutes. Add the farro and stir until coated, then slowly add the warm broth 1 cup at a time, constantly stirring until the liquid is absorbed. Continue to add broth until the farro is cooked, about 15 minutes. Stir in the butter and Parmesan cheese. Season to taste with salt and pepper. Serve immediately.   SERVES 6

forbidden rice

HEALTHY FATS, VEGETABLES, CARBOHYDRATES

LEVEL 1, LEVEL 2

Prepare the rice according to the package directions. Place in a mixing bowl and add the other ingredients. Mix well. Season with salt and pepper. Serve at room temperature. MAKES 3 CUPS OR 6 SERVINGS

1 cup uncooked
   Forbidden rice
   (Chinese black rice)

½ red onion, finely
   diced

1 bunch flat-leaf parsley,
   finely chopped

Zest and juice from
   1 lemon

¼ cup extra virgin olive
   oil

1 tablespoon chopped
   fresh mint leaves

Sea salt and freshly
   ground black pepper

fried rice with shiitake mushrooms

VEGETABLES , CARBOHYDRATES

LEVEL 1, LEVEL 2

Soak the dried mushrooms in 2 cups of warm water.

Place a large skillet over medium-high heat and add 2 tablespoons water. Add the shallot and sauté until tender, 3 minutes. Add the rices and stir together. Drain the mushrooms and coarsely chop, then add to the skillet along with the vegetable stock. Bring to a boil, then lower the heat and cover. Simmer for 25 minutes.

Add the vinegar and peas. Cover and simmer for another 5 minutes. SERVES 4

¼ cup dried shiitake
   mushrooms

1 shallot, minced

¼ cup uncooked wild
   rice

¼ cup uncooked brown
   rice

2 cups vegetable
   stock, preferably
   homemade
   (page 33)

1 tablespoon balsamic
   vinegar

½ cup frozen baby
   peas

red rice

2 tablespoons extra virgin olive oil

2 garlic cloves, finely chopped

2 shallots, finely chopped

1 medium zucchini, diced

1 medium yellow squash, diced

3 cups cooked red rice (or any whole-grain rice)

1 ripe medium tomato, seeded and diced

1 tablespoon finely chopped fresh chives, or 1 teaspoon dried

1 tablespoon julienned fresh basil leaves

1 scallion, white and green parts, finely sliced

Sea salt and freshly ground black pepper

Juice from ½ lemon

Heat a large sauté pan over medium heat. Add 1 tablespoon of the olive oil, the garlic, and the shallots. Sauté until soft, about 4 minutes. Add the zucchini and squash. Sauté until just cooked through, about 2 minutes. Add the cooked rice, tomato, chives, basil, and scallion. Season with salt and pepper, the lemon juice, and the remaining 1 tablespoon of olive oil. Serve hot or cold. SERVES 6

sautéed herb quinoa

HEALTHY FATS, VEGETABLES, CARBOHYDRATES
LEVEL 1, LEVEL 2

Prepare the quinoa according to package instructions.

While the quinoa is cooking, place a large sauté pan over medium heat. Add the olive oil and shallots; sauté for 2 minutes. Add the garlic and cook for 1 minute longer. When ready, add the cooked quinoa and the parsley, and stir to combine. Season with salt and pepper and serve immediately.   MAKES 3 CUPS OR 6 SERVINGS

1 cup dry quinoa

2 tablespoons extra virgin olive oil

2 shallots, finely diced

1 garlic clove, minced

2 teaspoons finely chopped flat-leaf parsley

Sea salt and freshly ground black pepper

quinoa tabbouleh

HEALTHY FATS, VEGETABLES, CARBOHYDRATES
LEVEL 1, LEVEL 2

In a medium bowl, combine the quinoa with all the other ingredients and season to taste with salt and pepper. Serve immediately. (The tabbouleh can be stored in an airtight container in the refrigerator for up to 1 week.)   MAKES 2 CUPS OR 4 SERVINGS

1 cup cooked quinoa

3 tablespoons extra virgin olive oil

1 cup chopped flat-leaf parsley

1/4 cup finely chopped shallots, or 1/4 red onion, minced

1 tablespoon chopped fresh dill, or 1/2 tablespoon dried dill weed

1 cup diced ripe tomato

1/2 cucumber, peeled, seeded, and diced

1 tablespoon chopped fresh mint leaves

Zest and juice from 1 lemon

Sea salt and freshly ground black pepper

tabbouleh

1 cup bulgur wheat

1¹/₂ cups vegetable
stock, preferably
homemade
(page 33)

2 garlic cloves, minced

2 tablespoons fresh
lemon juice

1 scallion, white and
green parts, sliced

¹/₄ cup chopped flat-
leaf parsley

Sea salt and freshly
ground black pepper

Place the bulgur in a large mixing bowl.

In a medium saucepan, bring the stock and garlic to a boil. Pour the hot stock over the bulgur. Stir, cover with a lid, and let the bulgur stand for 30 minutes. Mix in the remaining ingredients and season to taste with salt and pepper. SERVES 4

white bean salad with sage and thyme

1¹/₂ cups (1 pound)
dried small white
beans (navy,
cannellini, or
toscanelli)

1 yellow onion, halved

3 dried bay leaves

4 garlic cloves, crushed

1 celery stalk, chopped
into 2 pieces

1 sprig fresh sage

1 sprig fresh thyme

¹/₂ cup extra virgin olive
oil

3 tablespoons chopped
fresh thyme leaves,
or 1¹/₂ teaspoons
dried

1 red onion, finely
chopped

Sea salt and freshly
ground black pepper

Rinse the beans, picking them over to remove any debris. Place them in a large bowl with enough water to cover by 2 inches. Let soak overnight. (For a faster soak, add boiling water to cover and set aside for 1 hour.) Drain the beans, discarding the water.

Place the drained beans in a large saucepan and add cold water to cover by 1 inch. Add the onion, bay leaves, garlic, celery, sage and thyme sprigs, and 2 tablespoons of the oil. Cover and bring to a boil over medium heat, then reduce and simmer for about 1 hour. Add more water if the liquid is drying out. The beans are done when they are still slightly firm but not mushy.

Drain the beans and discard the vegetables and herb sprigs. Transfer to a large bowl. While still warm, toss with the thyme and red onion. Season to taste with salt and pepper and add the remaining 6 tablespoons olive oil. Serve immediately or reserve in the refrigerator. Bring to room temperature before serving. SERVES 8 TO 10

white bean garden salad

HEALTHY FATS, CARBOHYDRATES

LEVEL 1, LEVEL 2

Place the beans in a large, wide serving dish and toss with the olive oil, garlic, lemon juice, salt, and pepper. Proceed as if planting a beautiful garden. Take a large handful of the radish sprouts and insert them into the beans as if they grew out of them. Then repeat the process with a handful of fresh mint, again placing it into the beans as if it sprouted from them.

Arrange the tomatoes on a separate area of the beans. Place the capers in a mound in another area. Place the red onion in yet another area. Finally, sprinkle the feta around. The end result should look like a beautiful potted garden. Make sure to include a taste of all the elements when you serve. Season with additional salt and pepper.   SERVES 8

4 cups cooked white beans (cannellini or small white navy beans)

1/4 cup extra virgin olive oil

3 garlic cloves, minced

Juice from 1 lemon

Sea salt and freshly ground black pepper

1/2 pint radish sprouts

1 bunch fresh mint

2 ripe medium tomatoes, diced

2 tablespoons drained capers

1/2 red onion, coarsely chopped

8 ounces crumbled feta cheese

baby black lentil salad

HEALTHY FATS, CARBOHYDRATES

LEVEL 1, LEVEL 2

4 cups cooked baby
black lentils (or any
other lentils), cooled

2 shallots, finely diced

1 cucumber, peeled,
seeded, and diced

1 ripe tomato, seeded
and diced

2 scallions, white and
green parts, sliced

1 tablespoon julienned
fresh mint leaves,
plus extra for
garnish

Juice from $1/2$ lime

2 tablespoons extra
virgin olive oil

Sea salt and freshly
ground black pepper

Combine all the ingredients in a mixing bowl. Gently toss until the lentils are well coated. Adjust the seasonings with salt and pepper and additional lime juice. Garnish with mint and serve.   SERVES 8

french lentils

Place a large saucepan on low heat. Add the oil, celery, onion, and garlic. Sauté the vegetables for about 10 minutes, until they become soft. Add the lentils and stir to coat with the oil. Turn the heat up to medium and add the wine. Continue cooking until the wine reduces by half. Add 3 cups of the broth and bring to a boil, then reduce the heat and let simmer for 20 to 30 minutes, checking frequently to make sure the liquid does not completely evaporate. (Add more broth as needed.) Season with salt and pepper. Garnish with parsley and a squeeze of lemon juice. Serve warm or cold. MAKES 2 CUPS OR 4 SERVINGS

1 tablespoon extra virgin olive oil

1 celery stalk, very finely diced

$^1/_2$ yellow onion, very finely diced

2 garlic cloves

1 cup French de Puy lentils (or any other dried lentils)

$^1/_2$ cup dry white wine

3 to 4 cups chicken stock or broth, preferably homemade (pages 30–32)

Sea salt and freshly ground black pepper

1 tablespoon finely chopped flat-leaf parsley, for garnish

Juice from $^1/_2$ lemon, for garnish

black bean chili with spicy tomato salsa

VEGETABLES , CARBOHYDRATES

DETOX, LEVEL 1, LEVEL 2

BLACK BEAN CHILI

1 pound dried black beans, soaked overnight and drained, or fresh black shell beans

1 medium onion, diced

3 garlic cloves, minced

4 serrano chiles, finely chopped (see Note, page 39)

Sea salt and freshly ground black pepper

SPICY TOMATO SALSA

4 medium tomatoes, diced

1/2 medium cucumber, diced

1 bunch cilantro, coarsely chopped

1 red onion, diced

2 serrano chiles, finely chopped (see Note, page 39)

1 garlic clove, minced

Juice from 2 limes

For the chili: Place the beans in a large stockpot. Add water until the level is 2 inches above the beans. Add the onion, garlic, and chiles. Turn the heat to high. As the beans heat up, skim the foam off the top. When the beans come to a boil, turn the heat to low and simmer until tender, about 1 hour. Season with salt and pepper.

For the salsa: Gently combine all the salsa ingredients in a glass or other nonreactive bowl and set aside for the flavors to combine, about 30 minutes.

Serve the chili in bowls with a large spoonful of salsa.   SERVES 6

poultry

weeknight staples

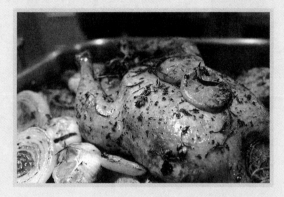

Out of all the recipes in this book, when it came to selecting one for the cover shot, I went for my ultimate signature dish, Zannie's Lemon Herb Chicken (page 205). On Sunday nights, when I can gather my brood, I like to have the family over for dinner, and I almost always serve chicken. I have to say, in my circle of family and friends, I'm kind of known for it. My family will tell you—of all my jobs, they think I am best at making chicken. That's a high compliment! I guess it started because Alan's son, Stephen, doesn't eat red meat, so chicken became the one dish that pleases everyone. And there are so many ways to prepare it, which is good, as often we eat it several nights a week.

Poultry is like the mushroom of the meat world; it takes on whatever flavors you add to it. My favorite seasonings are lemon, olive oil, onions, garlic, fresh tarragon, thyme, rosemary, and a generous coating of sea salt and pepper. Alan likes the legs roasted and crispy. My cool stepdaughter, Leslie, loves the Tuscan Flattened Chicken (page 211). Bruce likes it pounded thin, like my Chicken Piccata (page 219) or the Turkey Prosciutto with

Port Glaze (page 229). And all the grandkids go nuts for my Thanksgiving Turkey with Mushroom Sausage Stuffing and Tarragon Gravy (page 226) and also my Chicken Pot Pie (page 224)!

When I first started these books, my daughter-in-law, Caroline, said to me, "You have to teach people to make their chicken at home taste like yours." So I'll remind you: it's all in the quality of your ingredients! Purchase the best-quality food you can afford. The fresher, the better; the closer to its original source, the better; the more naturally it's raised, the better. And again, buy organic if you can.

Poultry is the ultimate mom food. Every bite tells my family they are loved. It's comfort food. It's nurturing. It's nutritious. There is no better meal, or job, on the planet.

zannie's lemon herb chicken

PROTEIN, HEALTHY FATS, VEGETABLES

DETOX, LEVEL 1, LEVEL 2

Preheat oven to 350°F.

Remove the giblets from the chicken. Rinse the bird and pat it dry. Place the chicken in a large roasting pan. Drizzle it with 2 tablespoons of the olive oil. Slice the tops off the garlic. Take one head and rub it all over the skin of the chicken, then place it in the cavity. Slice one of the lemons in half. Squeeze the juice from both halves over the chicken, then place the halves in the cavity. Liberally season the bird with salt and pepper. Add another drizzle of oil to the bottom of the pan, then add the onions and the remaining heads of garlic. Cover the chicken with the fresh herbs, and place a few of the herbs into the cavity. Slice the remaining lemons into ¼-inch-thick slices and place around the pan, with a few on top of the bird. Dot the bird with the butter.

Roast for 20 minutes per pound, approximately 2 hours. Carve the chicken and serve with the browned onions, baked garlic, lemon slices, crispy herbs, and a spoonful of drippings from the bottom of the pan. (*See color insert.*)   SERVES 4 TO 6

One 5- to 6-pound
    roasting chicken

3 tablespoons olive oil

4 heads garlic

4 lemons

Sea salt and freshly
    ground black pepper

3 onions, peeled and
    halved

1 bunch fresh tarragon,
    stems removed

1 bunch fresh sage,
    stems removed

1 bunch fresh rosemary,
    stems removed

1 bunch fresh thyme,
    stems removed

2 tablespoons unsalted
    butter

roast chicken with mushroom sausage stuffing and tarragon gravy

PROTEIN, HEALTHY FATS, VEGETABLES

DETOX, LEVEL 1, LEVEL 2

CHICKEN

One 5- to 6-pound roasting chicken

6 cups Mushroom Sausage Stuffing (page 227)

2 tablespoons olive oil

2 bunches fresh tarragon, stems removed

Sea salt and freshly ground black pepper

3 cups chicken stock or broth, preferably homemade (pages 30–32)

TARRAGON GRAVY

2 to 3 tablespoons pan drippings

2 cups dry white wine (use stock for Detox)

2 tablespoons unsalted butter

Preheat the oven to 350°F.

For the chicken: Remove the giblets from the chicken. Rinse the bird and pat it dry. Place as much of the stuffing as will fit into the cavity of the chicken. Rub the outside of the chicken with the olive oil, liberal amounts of tarragon, and salt and pepper. Pour the chicken stock into the bottom of a roasting pan. Add the chicken. Place a foil tent loosely over the chicken and bake for 1 hour, then remove the foil and cook for approximately 1 hour more (see Note).

Remove the cooked chicken and set aside. Pour off most of the fat in the pan, leaving 2 to 3 tablespoons to make the gravy.

For the gravy: Place the pan with the drippings on the stovetop over high heat. Add the wine and stir, constantly scraping the bottom of the pan to incorporate the browned bits. When the liquid is reduced by half, lower the heat and add the butter, 1 tablespoon at a time, until well combined.

Remove the stuffing from the chicken, carve, then serve with the gravy. SERVES 4 TO 6

NOTE An unstuffed chicken takes 20 minutes per pound to cook. Allow 25 minutes per pound for a stuffed chicken. The chicken is done when you prick the thigh with a fork and the juices run clear.

roasted herbes de provence chicken

PROTEIN, HEALTHY FATS, VEGETABLES, INSULIN TRIGGERS
DETOX, LEVEL 1, LEVEL 2

One 5- to 6-pound
roasting chicken

2 to 3 tablespoons olive
oil

Sea salt and freshly
ground black pepper

3 tablespoons herbes
de Provence

1 large bunch fresh
tarragon

3 yellow onions,
roughly chopped

2 carrots, peeled and
roughly chopped
(omit for Detox and
Level 1)

1 cup chicken stock or
broth, preferably
homemade
(pages 30–32)

1 cup dry white wine
(use stock for Detox)

1 tablespoon unsalted
butter

Preheat the oven to 350°F.

Remove the giblets from the chicken. Rinse the bird and pat it dry. Place it in a roasting pan and rub with some of the olive oil. Season with salt, pepper, and herbes de Provence. Place the tarragon under the skin, in the cavity, and all around the outside of the bird. Place one of the chopped onions in the cavity. Sprinkle the remaining onions and parsnips around the chicken in the pan.

Drizzle a little more oil on the vegetables. Pour the stock into the bottom of the pan. Put a foil tent on top of the chicken, and bake for 1 hour. Remove the tent and let brown for another hour (see Note, page 206).

Remove the chicken from the roasting pan and place it on a serving platter. Pour off most of the fat from the pan, reserving 2 to 3 table-spoons. Place the roasting pan on the stove and heat the drippings over high heat. Add the wine and scrape the browned bits off the bottom of the pan to make a sauce. Reduce for 5 to 7 minutes, or until desired thickness is achieved. Adjust seasonings to taste with salt and pepper. Turn off the heat and add the butter. Stir until well combined. Carve the chicken and serve with a spoonful of sauce. SERVES 4 TO 6

chicken with forty cloves of garlic

PROTEIN, HEALTHY FATS, VEGETABLES, INSULIN TRIGGERS

DETOX, LEVEL 1, LEVEL 2

One 5-pound roasting chicken

6 tablespoons olive oil

Sea salt and freshly ground black pepper

3 sprigs fresh thyme

2 sprigs fresh rosemary

3 sprigs fresh sage

40 garlic cloves, unpeeled

3 sprigs flat-leaf parsley

10 black peppercorns

1 cup chicken stock or broth, preferably homemade (pages 30–32), or more as needed

1 cup dry white wine (use stock for Detox)

Preheat the oven to 400°F.

Remove the giblets from the chicken. Rinse the bird and pat it dry. Rub the outside of the chicken with some of the olive oil. Season inside and out with salt and pepper. Put half the thyme, rosemary, and sage, plus 5 garlic cloves in the cavity of the chicken. Place the chicken in a Dutch oven fitted with a lid (or use a roasting pan and later cover tightly with foil). Scatter the remaining thyme, rosemary, sage, and garlic, and the parsley and peppercorns around the bird. Drizzle with the remaining olive oil. Pour the stock into the bottom of the pan. Cover and bake for approximately 1 hour, then remove the cover or foil and let the bird brown for another hour (see Note, page 206).

Remove the chicken from the pan and place it on a serving platter with the garlic spread all around. Put the pan with the drippings on the stovetop over high heat. Add the wine and scrape up any browned bits from the bottom of the pan, stirring constantly to reduce the sauce until it starts to thicken. If most of the drippings have evaporated, add another ½ cup of broth and reduce. Adjust salt and pepper to taste.

Carve the meat and serve with a spoonful of sauce and a few cloves of garlic. The garlic will easily slip out of the skins and add a delicious flavor to the chicken.   SERVES 4

tuscan flattened chicken

PROTEIN, HEALTHY FATS, VEGETABLES

DETOX, LEVEL 1, LEVEL 2

Season both sides of the chicken with salt, pepper, paprika, and rosemary. Heat the oil in an oversize skillet on medium-high heat. When the oil is hot, place the chicken, skin side down, into the skillet. Put a lid that is smaller than the skillet over the chicken, then weight it with a heavy stone or brick.

Cook for about 15 minutes, until the skin is golden brown. Remove the weight and the lid. Turn over the bird and replace the lid and weight. Cook for another 12 minutes. Chicken is done when the juices run clear.

Let chicken rest for about 10 minutes, then carve and serve. Garnish with rosemary sprigs.   SERVES 4

NOTE Have your butcher butterfly the chicken by cracking the breastbone so it will lie flat in the roasting pan.

One 4-pound chicken, butterflied (see Note)

Sea salt and freshly ground black pepper

Paprika

2 tablespoons chopped fresh rosemary, or 1 tablespoon dried

^{3}/4 cup olive oil

6 sprigs fresh rosemary, for garnish

farm-raised chicken st.-germain-beaupré with mushroom shallot dressing

CHICKEN

One 5- to 7-pound
roasting chicken

Sea salt

3 tablespoons olive oil

Freshly ground black
pepper

4 to 6 fresh tarragon
sprigs, or 2
tablespoons dried

1 tablespoon herbes de
Provence

3 tablespoons unsalted
butter

3 onions, quartered

PAN DRIPPINGS

2 cups boiling chicken
water

2 tablespoons (¼ stick)
unsalted butter

Sea salt and freshly
ground black pepper

Mushroom-Shallot
Dressing (recipe
follows)

Preheat the oven to 350°F.

For the chicken: Remove the giblets from the chicken. Rinse the bird and pat it dry. Fill your largest stockpot halfway with water and add 1 teaspoon of salt. Bring to a boil. Add the chicken and cover. Continue boiling on the stovetop for 20 to 25 minutes. Carefully lift out the chicken and reserve 2 cups of the water.

Place the parboiled chicken in a large roasting pan. Brush the outside of the chicken with some of the olive oil, salt, pepper, tarragon (place 1 tarragon sprig inside the cavity), and herbes de Provence. Dot the chicken all over with pats of butter. Rub the quartered onions with the remaining olive oil and place around the chicken in the roasting pan.

Place the pan in the hot oven for 35 to 40 minutes, basting often with pan juices. The bird is done when the skin is crispy brown and crackling and the leg jiggles back and forth easily. Remove from the oven and reserve the pan juices. Place the chicken on a platter. Leave the onions in the roasting pan. You do not have to pour the fat off from the pan because most of the fat was removed during the boiling process.

For the drippings: Put the roasting pan on the stove over high heat. Pour in the 2 cups reserved boiling chicken water and bring to a boil. Scrape the browned bits off the bottom of the pan to release the flavor. Reduce the sauce by one half. Turn off the heat. Add the butter, 1 tablespoon at a time, swirling until melted. Add salt and pepper to taste. Carve the chicken. Serve with the mushroom-shallot dressing and a spoonful of sauce. SERVES 4 TO 6

mushroom-shallot dressing

HEALTHY FATS, VEGETABLES, INSULIN TRIGGERS
DETOX, LEVEL 1, LEVEL 2

2 tablespoons olive oil

10 whole shallots, minced

1 pound mushrooms (any variety), chopped

Salt and freshly ground black pepper

2 tablespoons fresh tarragon leaves, or 1 tablespoon dried

$^1/_2$ cup dry white wine (use chicken stock for Detox)

2 tablespoons ($^1/_4$ stick) unsalted butter

Heat a skillet over medium heat. Add the olive oil. When the oil is just getting hot, add the shallots, stirring constantly so they brown but do not burn, 5 to 7 minutes. Add the mushrooms, turning often until they become soft and crusty on the edges, 10 to 15 minutes. Season with salt and pepper and tarragon.

Turn the heat up to high and add the wine or stock. Let the wine cook off for a couple of minutes, scraping the bits from the bottom of the pan. Then lower the heat and simmer for another 10 minutes. Turn off the heat and add the butter, 1 tablespoon at a time, stirring until the butter is melted and the mushrooms are coated. Store in an airtight container in the refrigerator for 1 to 2 weeks. MAKES 4 CUPS

balsamic roast chicken

PROTEIN, HEALTHY FATS, VEGETABLES, INSULIN TRIGGERS

DETOX, LEVEL 1, LEVEL 2

One 5- to 6-pound
roasting chicken

2 tablespoons chopped
fresh rosemary
leaves

2 tablespoons sea salt

3 garlic cloves,
chopped

1 tablespoon freshly
ground black pepper

2 red onions, chopped

¼ cup balsamic
vinegar

¼ cup dry red wine
(use chicken stock
for Detox)

Preheat the oven to 350°F.

To clean the chicken, remove any fatty pieces. Pull out the neck, giblets, and liver and reserve. Rinse the bird and pat it dry.

In a small dish, combine the rosemary, sea salt, garlic, and pepper. Rub this mixture all over the raw chicken inside and out. Let sit for at least 1 hour. (Can be prepared up to 24 hours in advance for flavors to take hold. Cover the chicken and place in the refrigerator.)

Place the neck, giblets, and liver on the bottom of a roasting pan. Sprinkle the chopped onions on top. Then place the whole chicken on top of the onions. Pour the balsamic vinegar and wine over the chicken.

Roast the chicken in the oven for approximately 2 hours (see Note, page 206).

Carve the chicken and serve with the balsamic and onion mixture from the bottom of the pan.   SERVES 4 TO 6

butterflied chicken with zucchini-ricotta stuffing

PROTEIN, HEALTHY FATS, VEGETABLES, CARBOHYDRATES
LEVEL 1, LEVEL 2

Clean the chicken thoroughly and pat it dry. Lay the chicken flat in the roasting pan. Gently separate the skin of the chicken with your hand, starting at the neck. Put your hand between the skin and the chicken meat and keep separating until the skin is loosened all the way to the bottom of the legs.

Shred the zucchini by grating it with the large circular holes of a grater. Place the shredded zucchini in a colander, toss with 2 tablespoons of salt, and let sit for 20 minutes. During this time, periodically pick up the shredded zucchini with your hands and squeeze it to remove the excess water. Rinse zucchini to remove the salt, and squeeze the water out one last time.

Preheat the oven to 350°F.

Place a small skillet over medium heat. Add the olive oil and garlic. Sauté the garlic until golden, about 1 minute.

In a bowl, combine the zucchini, sautéed garlic, ricotta, and salt and pepper to taste. Using your hands, mix the ingredients thoroughly. Stuff the zucchini-ricotta mixture *under* the skin of the chicken all the way down to the legs. Rub the skin with olive oil, salt, pepper, and herbes de Provence. Dot with butter.

Bake for about 2 hours. To carve, cut off leg and thigh pieces whole. Cut off wings. Slice the breast meat into large pieces to keep the stuffing intact. SERVES 4 TO 6

One 6-pound roasting chicken, butterflied (see Note, page 209)

4 zucchini, up to 1½ inches thick

Sea salt

2 tablespoons olive oil, plus extra for rubbing

3 garlic cloves, minced

One 15-ounce carton whole-milk ricotta cheese

Freshly ground black pepper

1 tablespoon herbes de Provence

2 tablespoons (¼ stick) unsalted butter

chicken breast with herbed goat cheese and wild mushroom sauce

PROTEIN, HEALTHY FATS, VEGETABLES

DETOX, LEVEL 1, LEVEL 2

3 ounces goat cheese

2 teaspoons chopped fresh thyme, or ½ teaspoon dried

2 teaspoons chopped flat-leaf parsley, or ½ teaspoon dried

2 teaspoons chopped fresh marjoram, or ½ teaspoon dried

2 chicken breasts (preferably airline cut; see Note)

Sea salt and freshly ground black pepper

Extra virgin olive oil

Wild Mushroom Sauce (recipe follows)

In a bowl, mix the goat cheese with the herbs. Making sure to keep the skin attached on one side, separate the skin from the chicken breasts to create a pocket. Fill each cavity with half the cheese mixture and press down on the skin to evenly distribute. Season the outside of both chicken breasts with salt and pepper.

Preheat the oven to 450°F.

Heat a large sauté pan (with an ovenproof handle) on medium-high. When the pan is hot, add 2 to 3 tablespoons of olive oil, and then add the chicken, skin side down. Sear the chicken for 3 minutes to get a brown, crispy skin. Using a wide spatula, gently turn the chicken (so as not to tear the skin) and continue cooking for another 3 minutes.

Place the sauté pan into the oven and roast chicken for 10 to 12 minutes. (If your sauté pan does not have an ovenproof handle, transfer to a casserole dish or roasting pan.) When the chicken is done, remove from the oven and place each breast onto a serving plate. Spoon the wild mushroom sauce over each chicken breast and serve immediately. SERVES 2

NOTE "Airline" breast refers to a chicken breast with the breastbone removed but the wing bone attached. Ask your butcher to do this for you, making sure to keep the skin attached. If you can't get this cut, use a boneless breast with the skin attached.

wild mushroom sauce

PROTEIN, HEALTHY FATS, VEGETABLES
DETOX, LEVEL 1, LEVEL 2

1 tablespoon extra virgin olive oil

1 garlic clove

1 cup fresh wild mushrooms

2 sprigs fresh thyme, leaves only, or $^1/_4$ teaspoon dried

$^1/_4$ cup dry white wine (use stock for Detox)

$^1/_2$ cup chicken stock or broth, preferably homemade (pages 30–32)

1 tablespoon veal or chicken demi-glace (optional)

1 tablespoon unsalted butter

Sea salt and freshly ground black pepper

Place a sauté pan on medium heat. Add the olive oil and the whole clove of garlic to infuse the flavor into the oil. Sauté the garlic for about 1 minute, and then add the mushrooms and thyme. Sauté until the mushrooms are crusty and golden brown, 10 to 15 minutes. Add the wine to deglaze the pan, scraping the browned bits from the bottom of the pan to release the flavor. Continue cooking until the wine reduces by half. Add the chicken broth and demi-glace, if using, and reduce again by half. Whisk in the butter and remove from the heat. Season with salt and pepper and serve as desired.   MAKES 1$^1/_2$ CUPS

clay pot chicken and leeks

PROTEIN, HEALTHY FATS, VEGETABLES

DETOX, LEVEL 1, LEVEL 2

4 large leeks, washed and halved, green tops removed

One 8-pound chicken, cut into pieces with skin removed

3 tablespoons ground cumin

Sea salt and freshly ground black pepper

3 tablespoons unsalted butter

3 cups chicken stock or broth, preferably homemade (pages 30–32)

If you have a clay pot, soak it in water overnight (or for at least 1 hour). If you don't have a clay pot, use a Dutch oven.

Preheat the oven to 325°F.

Line the bottom of the pot or Dutch oven with a third of the leeks. Then make a layer with half of the chicken. Sprinkle half of the cumin, salt, and pepper over the chicken. Dot with a tablespoon of butter.

Begin layering again with another third of the leeks and the remaining chicken, cumin, salt, pepper, and butter. Over the top layer, put an additional layer of leeks. Pour in the stock. Cover and bake for 2 hours or until chicken is cooked through. Serve chicken pieces in shallow bowls with spoonfuls of the sauce and leeks. SERVES 4

lemon roasted chicken

PROTEIN, HEALTHY FATS, VEGETABLES

DETOX, LEVEL 1, LEVEL 2

6 chicken legs, thighs attached (about 3 pounds)

2 medium yellow or sweet (Vidalia or Maui) onions, quartered

6 lemons

10 garlic cloves, pressed

1 tablespoon dried rosemary

$^1/_2$ teaspoon cayenne

Sea salt and freshly ground black pepper

Preheat the oven to 300°F.

Skin the chicken, if you like. Place the legs in a roasting pan with the quartered onions. Squeeze the juice from the lemons all over the chicken and then rub the pieces with garlic. Sprinkle on the rosemary, cayenne, salt, and pepper. Roast for about 90 minutes, or until cooked through.

To serve, pour the lemony garlic juices over the chicken and onions. SERVES 6

moroccan chicken with preserved lemon rinds

PROTEIN, HEALTHY FATS, VEGETABLES

DETOX, LEVEL 1, LEVEL 2

Heat the olive oil in a Dutch oven or a large pot with a lid. Add the chicken pieces and brown on both sides over high heat. Pour in 4 cups water. Add the garlic, onions, cilantro, parsley, cumin, ginger, saffron, and salt. Lower the heat, cover, and simmer for 1 hour.

Remove the chicken pieces, placing them on a platter. Turn the heat back up to high until the liquid boils and reduce liquid by one third. Add the preserved lemon rinds and olives and reduce the heat. Place the chicken pieces back in the sauce to reheat before serving.   SERVES 8

preserved lemon rinds

FREE FOOD

DETOX, LEVEL 1, LEVEL 2

Lemons
Kosher salt, 1 to 2 tablespoons per lemon
Water

1/4 cup olive oil

Two 3-pound chickens, skinned and cut into serving pieces

4 garlic cloves, minced

3 medium onions, coarsely chopped

1 cup chopped fresh cilantro

1 cup chopped flat-leaf parsley

4 teaspoons ground cumin

1 teaspoon ground ginger

1/2 teaspoon saffron

1/2 teaspoon sea salt

2 Preserved Lemon Rinds, thinly sliced (recipe follows)

1 cup red olives (for Level 1 and Level 2)

Thoroughly wash as many lemons as you care to make. Slice each lemon in half, lengthwise, from the stem side down to the bottom without cutting all the way through. Then slice again, from the stem almost down to the bottom, creating a quartered lemon that opens like a flower.

Pour the salt liberally inside each lemon. Gently close each lemon and place them in a clean jar with a lid that seals tightly. Fill the jar with as many lemons as will easily fit. Add water to the top of the jar, seal, and let sit for 30 days.

Remove the lemons one at a time. Scoop out the insides and discard. Slice the remaining lemon rind into desired sizes.

NOTE This simple process removes any bitterness from the lemon rind and creates a uniquely sweet yet tart flavor. They look beautiful displayed in glass jars on the kitchen counter.

chicken breasts stuffed with goat cheese–cilantro pesto

PROTEIN, HEALTHY FATS, VEGETABLES

DETOX, LEVEL 1, LEVEL 2

CHICKEN

Four 6-ounce boneless chicken breasts (with skin attached)

1/4 cup finely chopped cilantro leaves

1/4 cup chicken stock or broth, preferably homemade (pages 30–32)

2 tablespoons olive oil

Sea salt and freshly ground black pepper

STUFFING

2 garlic cloves

2 serrano chiles (see Note, page 39)

2 cups cilantro leaves

2 tablespoons olive oil

2 tablespoons freshly grated Parmesan cheese

3 ounces goat cheese

1/4 cup ricotta cheese

Sea salt and freshly ground black pepper

Heat a grill to medium high.

For the chicken: In a glass or other nonreactive container, place the chicken, cilantro leaves, stock, oil, and salt and pepper to taste. Marinate the breasts for 15 minutes, then drain, reserving the marinade.

Place the breasts on the grill, skin side down, and partially cook, 2 to 3 minutes per side, brushing frequently with the marinade. Remove and set aside. (Save the marinade.)

For the stuffing: In a blender or food processor, puree the garlic, chiles, cilantro, oil, and Parmesan, goat, and ricotta cheeses. Season with salt and pepper. Stuff this mixture under the skin of the chicken breasts, creating an even layer of stuffing. Place in the refrigerator until ready to use. (The chicken breasts can be prepared up to this point 6 hours before baking. Make sure to let them sit at room temperature for 15 minutes before baking.)

Preheat the oven to 375°F.

Place the breasts in a roasting pan and pour some of the reserved marinade over them. Bake for 12 minutes and serve immediately. SERVES 4

chicken piccata

PROTEIN, HEALTHY FATS, VEGETABLES, INSULIN TRIGGERS
DETOX, LEVEL 1, LEVEL 2

Two 6-ounce skinless
and boneless
chicken breasts (see
Note)

Sea salt and freshly
ground black pepper

2 tablespoons olive oil

$\frac{1}{4}$ cup dry white wine
(use chicken stock
for Detox)

2 tablespoons drained
capers

Juice from 1 lemon

1 tablespoon unsalted
butter

Rinse the chicken breasts and pat them dry. Place each breast flat on a chopping block. With your knife parallel to the chopping block, slice the breast in half through the middle to make it half as thick. Pound each half with a mallet until ¼ inch thick. Season each breast with salt and pepper.

Place a skillet over high heat, add the olive oil and as many of the chicken slices as will fit in the pan without overlapping. Brown for 2 minutes on each side, then set aside in a warm oven.

Reheat the skillet over medium heat. Add the wine and reduce for 2 minutes or so, stirring constantly to scrape the browned bits off the bottom of the pan. Stir in the capers and the lemon juice. Remove from heat and add the butter, stirring until melted. Adjust the salt and pepper to taste. Pour the sauce over the chicken and serve.   SERVES 2

NOTE If you prefer, ask your butcher to pound the chicken into four ¼-inch-thick cutlets.

chicken paillard with lemon-parsley butter and seared red chard

Two 6-ounce skinless and boneless chicken breasts (see Note, page 219)

Sea salt and freshly ground black pepper

4 tablespoons olive oil

6 tablespoons (³/4 stick) unsalted butter

10 shallots, finely diced

Juice from 3 lemons

¹/2 cup chicken stock or broth, preferably homemade (pages 30–32)

2 teaspoons chopped flat-leaf parsley

2 bunches red Swiss chard, coarsely chopped

Rinse the chicken breasts and pat them dry. Place each breast flat on a chopping block. With your knife parallel to the chopping block, slice the breast in half through the middle to make it half as thick. Pound each half with a mallet until ¼ inch thick. Season each breast with salt and pepper.

Heat a skillet over high heat. Add 3 tablespoons of the olive oil and as many of the chicken slices as will fit in the pan without overlapping. Brown for 2 minutes on each side, then set aside in a shallow baking pan in an oven on warm. Repeat with remaining chicken.

Place the chicken skillet over medium heat and melt 3 tablespoons of the butter. Add the shallots, cooking until soft, about 5 minutes. Add the lemon juice and chicken stock and bring to a boil. Scrape any bits off the bottom of the pan to release the flavor. Reduce the liquid by half. Cut the remaining 3 tablespoons butter into small pieces and whisk into the pan until the sauce is smooth. Remove from the heat. Stir in additional salt, pepper, and the parsley. Keep warm.

Heat a wok or large skillet over very high heat. Add the remaining tablespoon olive oil and the chard, quickly cooking until just wilted, about 1 minute. Season with salt and pepper. Arrange the chicken over the chard on a platter and top with the lemon-parsley butter.

SERVES 2

chicken paillard with fresh tomato salsa and arugula

PROTEIN, HEALTHY FATS, VEGETABLES
DETOX, LEVEL 1, LEVEL 2

For the salsa: Combine all the ingredients in a medium bowl and set aside to let the flavors combine. (Do not refrigerate or the tomatoes will get mealy.)

For the chicken: Rinse the chicken breasts and pat them dry. Place each breast flat on a chopping block. With your knife parallel to the chopping block, slice the breast in half through the middle to make it half as thick. Pound each half with a mallet until ¼ inch thick. Season each breast with salt, pepper, and rosemary.

Heat a skillet over high heat. Add the olive oil and as many of the chicken pieces as will fit in the pan without overlapping. Brown for 2 to 3 minutes on each side and set aside in an oven on warm. Repeat with the remaining chicken.

Line four dinner plates with fresh arugula. Arrange two pieces of chicken on top of the arugula on each plate and garnish each plate with a large spoonful of salsa.   SERVES 4

NOTE If you prefer, ask your butcher to pound the chicken into eight ¼-inch-thick cutlets.

SALSA
4 medium tomatoes, diced

1 bunch flat-leaf parsley, chopped

2 garlic cloves, minced

2 tablespoons extra virgin olive oil

Juice from ½ lemon

Sea salt and freshly ground black pepper

CHICKEN PAILLARD
Four 6-ounce skinless and boneless chicken breasts (see Note)

Sea salt and freshly ground black pepper

2 sprigs fresh rosemary, chopped, or 2 tablespoons dried

2 tablespoons olive oil

1 bunch fresh arugula (or your favorite green)

chicken breasts with sage

Four 6-ounce skinless
and boneless
chicken breasts

Sea salt and freshly
ground black pepper

Juice from 3 lemons

6 tablespoons olive oil

40 fresh sage leaves, or
2 teaspoons dried

4 tablespoons (1/2 stick)
unsalted butter

4 lemons wedges, for
garnish

Season the chicken breasts with salt and pepper. Place them in a casserole dish. Add the lemon juice, half of the oil, and the sage. Turn the chicken to coat evenly, cover, and set aside at room temperature for 30 minutes.

Heat a large skillet on medium heat. Add the butter and the remaining 3 tablespoons oil. When hot and bubbly, take each piece of chicken out of the marinade (reserving marinade and sage) and place in the skillet. Cook until golden brown, about 5 minutes. Turn the chicken breasts over, then remove the sage leaves from the marinade and add to the bottom of the skillet. Cook another 5 to 7 minutes, until breasts are cooked through. The sage should get crispy in the bottom of the pan. (If it is getting overcooked, remove it from the pan and set aside.) Remove the chicken breasts and sage and cover loosely with foil while you make the sauce.

Return the pan to medium-high heat. Add the reserved marinade and stir with a wooden spoon, scraping up the browned bits from the bottom of the pan. Let the sauce boil until it reduces to a thick syrupy sauce, about 1 minute. Pour the sauce over the chicken. Garnish with the lemon wedges. Serve immediately. SERVES 4

chicken scaloppine with tarragon

PROTEIN, HEALTHY FATS, VEGETABLES, INSULIN TRIGGERS
DETOX, LEVEL 1, LEVEL 2

Season both sides of the cutlets with salt and pepper. Place 1 large tarragon sprig on each piece of chicken. On top of the cutlet and tarragon, place 1 piece of pancetta. Press the tarragon and pancetta against the cutlet to make them stick. Repeat until all the cutlets are prepared. (The cutlets may be prepared as above up to 4 hours in advance. Cover them and place in the refrigerator. Just make sure you remove them from the refrigerator 15 minutes before cooking to allow them to come to room temperature.)

Place a large skillet over medium-high heat. Add the olive oil and 2 tablespoons of the butter. When the butter is melted, add as many cutlets as will fit flat in the pan. Cook for 2 minutes on each side. As the cutlets are cooked, set aside in a warm oven. Continue until all the cutlets are cooked.

After removing the last cutlets from the skillet, add the wine. Cook until the steam disappears. Add the stock, then reduce the sauce by half, turn off the heat, and stir in the remaining 1 tablespoon butter until melted.

Place two cutlets on each plate and top with a little sauce. Serve with a lemon wedge. SERVES 4

NOTE Ask your butcher to pound the cutlets to ¼-inch scaloppine.

8 chicken cutlets, pounded to $1/4$-inch thickness (see Note)

Sea salt and freshly ground black pepper

8 sprigs fresh tarragon

8 paper-thin slices pancetta (or prosciutto)

2 tablespoons olive oil

3 tablespoons unsalted butter

$1/2$ cup dry white wine (use stock for Detox)

$1/2$ cup chicken stock or broth, preferably homemade (pages 30–32)

4 lemon wedges, for serving

chicken pot pie

PROTEIN, HEALTHY FATS, CARBOHYDRATES, INSULIN TRIGGERS

LEVEL 2

6 tablespoons olive oil

Three 6-ounce skinless and boneless chicken breasts, cut into 1-inch fingers, or 3 cups cooked chicken

3 yellow onions, thinly sliced

1 garlic clove, chopped

2 red bell peppers, cored and thinly sliced, then cut in half

2 tablespoons (¼ stick) unsalted butter, plus ¼ cup (½ stick) melted

1 tablespoon whole wheat flour

2 cups chicken stock or broth, preferably homemade (pages 30–32)

¼ teaspoon red pepper flakes, or to taste

½ teaspoon sea salt

Freshly ground black pepper

1 package phyllo dough, thawed

Preheat the oven to 350°F.

Heat a medium sauté pan (with straight sides) on high heat. Add 2 tablespoons of the olive oil. If using raw chicken, sauté until browned and cooked through, about 5 minutes. Remove with a slotted spoon and reserve on a plate.

Adding more oil as needed, fry the sliced onions over medium heat for 15 minutes, until golden brown. Add the garlic and sauté for 2 minutes. Add the red peppers and sauté for 5 minutes more.

Add the 2 tablespoons butter and stir it into the mixture. Add the flour and cook for 2 minutes, stirring constantly. Then add the chicken stock, red pepper flakes, salt, and pepper. Reduce liquid for 5 minutes more. Add the chicken and cook for another 2 to 5 minutes. Sauce should be thickened and brown in color. Place the hot filling in a baking dish. (This recipe can be made in advance up to this point. Reheat the filling before assembling the phyllo crust.)

When you are ready to assemble the pie, brush 5 sheets of phyllo with melted butter and arrange the phyllo atop the filling one sheet at a time in a ruffled-flower free-form design.

Bake for 10 minutes. Watch carefully, as the crust should be lightly browned and crisp. Serve immediately. SERVES 4 TO 6

chicken curry with cucumber salad

PROTEIN, HEALTHY FATS, VEGETABLES
DETOX, LEVEL 1, LEVEL 2

Place the oil in a large skillet over medium-high heat. When hot, add the onion and sauté until translucent, about 4 minutes. Add the ginger and garlic and sauté for 2 minutes longer. Add the chicken and sauté approximately 4 minutes. Add the tomatoes with their juice, the cilantro, curry powder, cumin, chili powder, and salt and pepper to taste. Stir until the chicken is well coated with the spices.

Cover, lower the heat, and simmer for about 30 minutes. As it cooks, the juice from the tomatoes will be absorbed by the chicken. (If there is not enough liquid, add a little water.) After 30 minutes, if there is still liquid left in the pan, uncover it, turn up the heat to medium, and cook off the liquid. Serve with cucumber salad.   SERVES 4

cucumber salad

HEALTHY FATS, VEGETABLES
DETOX, LEVEL 1, LEVEL 2

2 cups crème fraîche (page 149) or nonfat yogurt

1 medium cucumber, peeled and thinly sliced

1 sweet onion (Vidalia or Maui), thinly sliced

Combine all the ingredients in a bowl. Chill and serve.   SERVES 4

---

2 tablespoons olive oil

1 medium onion, finely chopped

1 tablespoon grated fresh ginger

1 tablespoon minced garlic

Four 6-ounce skinless and boneless chicken breasts, chopped into bite-size pieces

2 tomatoes, finely chopped, with juice and seeds

1/2 cup cilantro, finely chopped

1 tablespoon garam masala (curry powder)

1 tablespoon ground cumin

1/2 teaspoon chili powder

Sea salt and freshly ground black pepper

Cucumber Salad (recipe follows)

chicken patty lemon piccata

PROTEIN, HEALTHY FATS
DETOX, LEVEL 1, LEVEL 2

2 pounds ground
  chicken

4 tablespoons olive oil

1/2 cup chicken stock
  or broth, preferably
  homemade
  (pages 30–32)

Sea salt and freshly
  ground black pepper

Juice from 1 lemon

4 tablespoons (1/2 stick)
  unsalted butter

1 lemon, sliced

Separate the ground chicken into patties and flatten them. In a heated skillet, add the olive oil and fry the patties until cooked and crusty, about 1½ minutes on each side. Remove the patties when cooked. Add the chicken stock to the skillet and scrape up all the browned bits from the bottom for about 3 minutes, or until the broth is reduced by half. Season with salt and pepper and the lemon juice. Turn off the heat and add the butter, stirring until the sauce is smooth. Pour over the chicken patties. Garnish with the lemon slices and serve immediately.

SERVES 4

thanksgiving turkey with mushroom sausage stuffing and tarragon gravy

PROTEIN, HEALTHY FATS, VEGETABLES
DETOX, LEVEL 1, LEVEL 2

One 14-pound turkey

6 cups Mushroom
  Sausage Stuffing
  (recipe follows)

6 tablespoons
  (3/4 stick) unsalted
  butter, softened

2 bunches fresh
  tarragon, chopped

Sea salt and freshly
  ground black pepper

8 cups chicken stock
  or broth, preferably
  homemade
  (pages 30–32)

Preheat the oven to 325°F.

Remove the giblets from the turkey. Rinse the bird and pat it dry. Fill the cavity of the turkey with the stuffing. Rub the outside of the turkey with 3 tablespoons of the butter, the tarragon, salt, and pepper. Pour 6 cups of the stock into the bottom of the roasting pan.

Bake the turkey for about 4 hours, basting every 30 minutes or so. If the bird starts getting too brown, cover with a foil tent. (Check for doneness with a meat thermometer—it should register somewhere between 162°F and 170°F.) When the turkey is cooked, remove it from the pan and keep warm.

Pour off all but 2 to 3 tablespoons of the fat in the roasting pan. Heat the remaining 2 cups stock. Place the roasting pan on the stovetop over high heat and add the hot stock, scraping the browned bits off the bottom of the pan. Reduce by half and remove from the heat. Add the remaining butter, 1 tablespoon at a time, until well combined.

Carve the turkey and serve with the stuffing and tarragon-flavored gravy.

SERVES 12 TO 14

mushroom sausage stuffing

PROTEIN, HEALTHY FATS, VEGETABLES, INSULIN TRIGGERS
DETOX, LEVEL 1, LEVEL 2

4 onions, thinly sliced

2 to 4 tablespoons olive oil

4 cups coarsely chopped fresh shiitake and oyster mushrooms, or white button mushrooms

Sea salt and freshly ground black pepper

1/2 cup dry white wine (use chicken stock for Detox)

2 tablespoons (1/4 stick) unsalted butter

2 pounds spicy turkey sausage, meat removed from casings

1 bunch fresh tarragon, leaves only

Sauté the onions in the olive oil over medium heat until caramelized, about 30 minutes. Turn the heat up to medium high and add the mushrooms. Sauté the mushrooms until crisp on the edges, 10 to 15 minutes. Season with salt and pepper. Turn the heat to high and add the wine. Let the wine cook off for a couple of minutes, then lower the heat and simmer with the mushrooms for another 10 minutes. Stir in the butter 1 tablespoon at a time until combined. Remove from the heat and set aside.

In a large skillet, brown the sausage. When cooked through, 5 to 7 minutes, add to the mushroom mixture along with the tarragon and combine thoroughly. MAKES 6 CUPS

roast turkey breast stuffed with prosciutto, fontina, and sage

PROTEIN, HEALTHY FATS, VEGETABLES, INSULIN TRIGGERS

DETOX, LEVEL 1, LEVEL 2

½ cup grated fontina cheese

½ cup julienned prosciutto

2 tablespoons julienned fresh sage

Sea salt and freshly ground black pepper

One 2-pound boneless turkey breast

Olive oil

1 cup dry white wine (or broth for Detox)

½ cup chicken stock or broth, preferably homemade (pages 30–32)

2 tablespoons (¼ stick) unsalted butter

Preheat the oven to 425°F.

In a small bowl, combine the cheese, prosciutto, and sage. Sprinkle with salt and pepper.

Create a pocket in the turkey breast to hold the stuffing by inserting a carving knife into the middle of the breast almost to the other side of the breast. Twist and turn until you create a cavity. Using your hand, insert the stuffing into the cavity. Season the turkey well with salt and pepper and drizzle with olive oil. Place in a roasting pan and put into the oven for 20 minutes. Lower the heat to 350°F and roast until done, approximately 45 minutes to an hour, or until the temperature reaches 165°F on a meat thermometer. Remove from the oven and allow to cool slightly.

Remove the turkey from the pan and place the pan on top of the stove. Over medium heat, add the wine and reduce by half, scraping the sides and bottom of the pan in order to get all the browned bits into the sauce. Add the stock and bring to a simmer, then add the butter. Adjust seasoning to taste.

Slice the turkey breast and place it on plates. Spoon the sauce over the turkey and serve immediately. SERVES 4

turkey prosciutto with port glaze

PROTEIN, HEALTHY FATS, VEGETABLES

LEVEL 1, LEVEL 2

12 turkey cutlets (breast slices), pounded to 1/4-inch thickness

Sea salt and freshly ground black pepper

24 fresh sage leaves, or 2 tablespoons ground

12 paper-thin slices prosciutto

3 tablespoons olive oil

3 tablespoons unsalted butter

1/2 cup port wine

Season both sides of the cutlets with salt and pepper. Place 2 sage leaves onto each piece of turkey. On top of the cutlet and sage, place 1 piece prosciutto. Press the sage and prosciutto against the cutlet to make them stick. Repeat until all the cutlets are prepared. (The cutlets may be prepared to this point up to 4 hours in advance. Cover them and place in the refrigerator. Just make sure you remove them from the refrigerator 15 minutes before cooking to let the meat come to room temperature.)

Put the olive oil and 2 tablespoons of butter in a large frying pan. When the butter is melted, add as many cutlets as will fit flat in the pan. Cook for 2 minutes on each side. As the cutlets are cooked, set them aside in a warm oven. Continue until all the cutlets are cooked.

After removing the last cutlets from the frying pan, add the port wine. Cook until the steam disappears. Reduce the sauce by half, then turn off the heat and stir in the remaining 1 tablespoon butter until melted.

Place two cutlets on each plate and top with a little sauce.   SERVES 6

turkey cutlets with classic marinara sauce

MARINARA SAUCE

2 tablespoons olive oil

1 medium onion, chopped

4 garlic cloves, pressed

One 28-ounce can tomato sauce

2 tablespoons chopped flat-leaf parsley

1 teaspoon dried basil

1/2 teaspoon dried oregano

TURKEY

4 turkey cutlets (breast slices), pounded to 1/4-inch thickness

1 tablespoon dried rosemary

1 teaspoon dried thyme

Sea salt and freshly ground black pepper

4 tablespoons olive oil

For the marinara sauce: Heat the olive oil in a saucepan. Add the onion and cook until translucent, approximately 5 minutes. Add the garlic and cook 1 minute longer. Add the tomato sauce and herbs and bring to a boil. Lower the heat and simmer for 1 hour or more.

For the turkey: Season the cutlets with the rosemary, thyme, salt, and pepper. Heat the olive oil in a large skillet over medium-high heat. Add the turkey cutlets—as many as will fit without overlapping. Brown the cutlets on both sides and continue cooking until cooked through, 2 to 3 minutes per side. Cover and keep warm. Repeat with remaining cutlets.

Serve the cutlets topped with marinara sauce.   SERVES 4

turkey sausages with peppers and onions

PROTEIN, HEALTHY FATS, VEGETABLES

DETOX, LEVEL 1, LEVEL 2

In a large sauté pan over medium heat, cook the onions and peppers in the olive oil, stirring frequently until the peppers are soft and the onions are caramelized, about 30 minutes. Cook the sausages on a grill or brown them in a skillet and serve them atop a heaping mound of peppers and onions. SERVES 6

2 large yellow or sweet (Vidalia or Maui) onions, thinly sliced

4 red, orange, or yellow bell peppers, cored, seeded, and julienned

¼ cup olive oil

12 hot Italian turkey sausages

turkey meatloaf

PROTEIN, HEALTHY FATS, VEGETABLES

DETOX, LEVEL 1, LEVEL 2

Preheat the oven to 350°F.

In a large mixing bowl, combine all the ingredients except the stock. Form into a loaf and place in a lightly greased loaf pan.

Pour the stock over the top and bake for 1 hour, basting periodically. When finished, cut into slices and spoon the juices from the bottom of the pan over the meat. SERVES 4

1 pound ground dark-meat turkey

1 large egg yolk

3 tablespoons chopped flat-leaf parsley

1 tablespoon unsalted butter, softened

½ medium onion, chopped

1 teaspoon fresh lemon juice

1 teaspoon sea salt

1 teaspoon freshly ground black pepper

1 cup chicken stock or broth, preferably homemade (pages 30–32)

confit of duck

8 duck legs

1 cup coarse kosher salt

2 tablespoons cracked black peppercorns

1/4 cup mixed dried herbs (thyme, marjoram, bay leaf)

1/2 tablespoon allspice berries, crushed

1/2 tablespoon juniper berries, crushed

6 cups rendered duck fat

6 garlic cloves

Rinse the duck pieces and pat dry. Combine the salt, pepper, herbs, and spices in a bowl. Coat each piece of duck in the mixture and lay flat in a dish, sprinkling the remainder of the salt mixture on top. Refrigerate for at least 2 hours (even better, up to 24 hours).

Wipe the duck pieces free of salt. Melt the rendered fat in a Dutch oven and put the duck pieces in it close together so that the duck is covered with the fat. Add the garlic and simmer very gently until the duck is tender, about 2 hours. When pierced with a fork, the duck should fall off the fork when shaken.

Transfer the duck to a baking dish and add the fat. (Try not to bring any juice with the duck.) The duck should be completely covered with the fat. It will stay preserved in the fat for up to 8 weeks in the refrigerator. To serve, lift the duck out of the fat, then remove and discard any skin or extra fat. Reheat in a 400°F oven for 15 minutes and serve immediately. SERVES 4

roast christmas goose with port glaze

PROTEIN, HEALTHY FATS, VEGETABLES, FRUIT

LEVEL 1, LEVEL 2

Preheat the oven to 350°F.

For the goose: Clean the goose thoroughly and remove any extra fatty pieces. Reserve the giblets for the sauce. Stuff the goose with the onion halves, fresh thyme, and salt and pepper. Rub the goose with olive oil. Season with about 1 tablespoon each of the salt, pepper, sage, dried thyme, poultry seasoning, and allspice. Prick the bird all over with a fork lightly to allow the excess fat to escape.

Roast the goose on a rack in a roasting pan for 20 to 25 minutes per pound, basting occasionally. The bird is done when the legs jiggle easily and the juices run clear when the skin is pierced.

For the glaze: While the goose is roasting, place the giblets, celery, garlic, onion, parsley, and 6 cups of water in a saucepan and bring to a boil. Reduce the heat and skim the foam off the top. Simmer for 2 hours. Strain, reserving the stock. Finely chop the giblets and set aside.

Remove the goose from the pan and skim almost all the fat from the juices with a large spoon. Place the roasting pan with goose drippings over medium heat. Scrape the browned bits from the bottom of the pan. Add the port, 2 cups of reserved stock, and the chopped giblets. Reduce over high heat, stirring for about 15 minutes, or until slightly thickened. Add the currants. Add salt and pepper to taste.

Pour the port glaze over the carved goose.   SERVES 4 TO 6

GOOSE

One 10- to 14-pound goose

1 onion, halved

2 teaspoons chopped fresh thyme leaves

Sea salt and freshly ground black pepper

3 tablespoons olive oil

1 tablespoon dried sage

1 tablespoon dried thyme

1 tablespoon poultry seasoning

1 tablespoon ground allspice

PORT GLAZE

Goose giblets (except the liver)

4 celery stalks

3 garlic cloves, peeled

1 large onion, chopped

4 sprigs flat-leaf parsley

1 cup port wine

14 ounces dried currants, soaked in water until soft and drained (omit for Level 1)

Sea salt and freshly ground black pepper

fish and seafood
fresh!

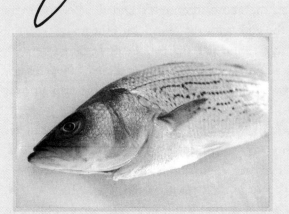

Thanksgiving is our family's biggest holiday. Odd opener for the Fish and Seafood chapter, right? Not if you are part of our annual Friday Crab Lunch in the desert!

The day after Thanksgiving, each and every year, we gather our friends and family at long tables outside on our deck. Each person is served a freshly cracked Dungeness crab, still warm and simply wrapped in butcher paper. The table is set with crab crackers, lemon wedges, Homemade Mayonnaise (page 148), and chilled Sonoma Cutrer Chardonnay. And for dessert I make my delicious Lemon Curd Tart (page 332). We all sit around cracking, laughing, and stuffing our faces with sweet, delectable crab! Being born and raised in San Francisco, I have always had access to crab. I didn't like it as a kid and used to give mine to my brother. Lucky Danny. Now I love it, and I have a lifetime of memories collected from this magical family tradition.

When fish and seafood are fresh, just pulled from the river or ocean, there is nothing like it. Again, extra virgin olive oil, lemon, herbs, sea salt, and butter are my preferred ingredients for seafood, as you'll find in my Pan-Fried Petrale Sole (page 243). When I was a young single mother, I could get two pieces of petrale sole inexpensively, so Bruce and I ate this often. If salmon is more to your taste, make sure to try Salmon Steaks with Fried Ginger and Lime (page 236). Or, try the Broiled Sea Bass with Candied Tomatoes and Seared Escarole (page 241).

The fish are jumpin'.

salmon steaks with fried ginger and lime

PROTEIN, HEALTHY FATS, VEGETABLES

DETOX, LEVEL 1, LEVEL 2

FRIED GINGER

One 3-inch piece fresh ginger

$1/2$ cup grapeseed oil

SALMON

Four 6-ounce salmon steaks

2 tablespoons olive oil

Sea salt and freshly ground black pepper

2 limes, 1 sliced paper-thin with peel and 1 juiced

2 Kirby cucumbers, halved lengthwise and thinly sliced

Handful of daikon sprouts (optional)

3 tablespoons soy sauce

For the ginger: Peel the ginger and thinly slice. Cut the slices into thin strips. Heat the oil in a frying pan. When hot, add the ginger and cook until dark golden brown. Remove with a slotted spoon; set aside to drain on paper towels.

For the salmon: Prepare and heat a grill to medium high. Brush the salmon steaks with a little olive oil, then season with salt and pepper. Grill until just cooked through; cooking time will vary depending on the thickness of the fish, from 2 to 7 minutes per side.

Cut each lime slice, including its rind, into 8 pieces, as if you were cutting a pie. Toss the lime with the cucumbers and daikon sprouts, if using. Mix the soy sauce and lime juice, and toss with the vegetables. Place the salmon on four individual plates and heap the vegetable garnish on the fish. Top with a sprinkle of fried ginger. SERVES 4

braised salmon in white wine and fresh ginger

PROTEIN, HEALTHY FATS, VEGETABLES, INSULIN TRIGGERS

LEVEL 1, LEVEL 2

1 bottle dry white wine

2 lemons

⅓ cup peeled and grated fresh ginger

One 8- to 10-pound whole salmon, cleaned but with skin, head, and tail left on

Sea salt and freshly ground black pepper

Fresh herbs, for garnish

Pour the wine into a fish poacher or a covered pan fitted with a rack. Squeeze the juice from 1 lemon into the wine and add the fresh ginger. Slice the other lemon and place in the cavity of the fish along with salt and pepper. Place the fish on the rack, not in the liquid. Cover and bring the liquid to a boil, steaming the fish for 15 minutes.

Lower the heat so the liquid is barely at a simmer. Steam the salmon for about 1½ hours, checking periodically that there is enough liquid in the pan. If necessary, add more wine. The salmon is cooked when a meat thermometer registers 150°F. Remove the rack from the poacher and place the fish on a serving platter. Quickly remove the skin from the top of the fish.

Reduce the pan juices over high heat until about 1 cup of thickened sauce remains. Spoon the delicious ginger-wine sauce over the fish. Garnish the platter with fresh herbs.   SERVES 12

crispy-skinned salmon with roasted garlic aïoli and warm radicchio–shiitake mushroom salad

PROTEIN, HEALTHY FATS, VEGETABLES

DETOX, LEVEL 1, LEVEL 2

Olive oil

Two 6-ounce salmon fillets, 1½ inches thick, with skin on

Sea salt and freshly ground black pepper

6 fresh shiitake mushrooms, stemmed and julienned

½ head radicchio

1 cup arugula, loosely packed

1 cup Roasted Garlic Aïoli (recipe follows)

Preheat the oven to 350°F.

Drizzle the olive oil over the salmon and season with salt and pepper. Heat a sauté pan on high, then add about 2 tablespoons olive oil. Add the salmon fillets and sear on each side for about 3 minutes. Place onto a serving dish and set aside to keep warm.

Add the mushrooms to the pan and toss over medium heat until crusty, about 5 minutes. Add the radicchio and arugula, and toss quickly for 15 seconds, or until just wilted. Season with salt and pepper.

Place the warm salad beside the salmon, then spoon the aïoli over the top of the fish. Serve immediately.   SERVES 2

roasted garlic aïoli

PROTEIN, HEALTHY FATS, VEGETABLES

DETOX, LEVEL 1, LEVEL 2

1 head garlic

1 large egg

1 large egg yolk

1 tablespoon Dijon mustard

Juice from $1/2$ lemon

1 cup light olive oil

Preheat the oven to 350°F.

Place the garlic in a baking dish and roast for about 45 minutes. Squeeze the garlic cloves from their skin and place into a blender or food processor with the egg, egg yolk, mustard, and lemon juice. Puree until smooth. Add the oil in a slow drizzle until the aïoli emulsifies. Store in an airtight container in the refrigerator for up to 1 week. MAKES 1 CUP

crispy mesquite salmon

One 2-pound fresh
salmon or trout fillet,
skin attached

1 cup cream

1 tablespoon black
peppercorns

1 tablespoon green
peppercorns

1 teaspoon coriander
seeds

1 teaspoon dill seed

Sea salt and freshly
ground black pepper

2 tablespoons
mayonnaise

1 teaspoon dried dill
weed

2 lemons, quartered

2 limes, quartered

Heat the grill to medium high. If you are using a gas grill, buy some mesquite chips and soak them in water for a few hours. Before you light the grill, place the chips around the briquettes.

Soak the fish in the cream for approximately 30 minutes. Meanwhile, crack the peppercorns and seeds using the bottom of a heavy skillet. Combine them with 2 teaspoons salt.

Remove the fish from the cream. Spread half the mayonnaise on the skin of the fish. Season with salt and pepper. Turn the fish over, exposing the flesh side. Spread the remaining mayonnaise over the flesh and sprinkle with the dill weed. Rub the seasonings into the flesh. All the flesh should be covered with the mayonnaise and seasonings.

Place the fish on the hot grill, seasoning side down. Cook for 5 to 7 minutes. Turn over with a spatula and grill the other side for an additional 7 minutes, or until the fish flakes when you touch it with a fork. (If you don't have a grill, cook it under the broiler.)

Remove the fish from the grill and place it on a platter, surrounded by lemon and lime wedges. SERVES 4

broiled sea bass with candied tomatoes and seared escarole

PROTEIN, HEALTHY FATS, VEGETABLES

DETOX, LEVEL 1, LEVEL 2

Preheat the broiler.

Brush the fish with a little olive oil and sprinkle with salt and pepper. Place the fish on a broiling pan and broil until golden brown and just cooked through the center, approximately 4 minutes per side. Cooking time will vary depending on the thickness of the fish.

Heat a large skillet or wok over high heat. Add a little olive oil and sauté the escarole until tender, about 4 minutes. Sprinkle with salt and pepper. Arrange on four plates. Place the sea bass on top of the escarole and top each piece of fish with 3 candied tomato halves.   SERVES 4

Four 6-ounce sea bass fillets

Olive oil

Sea salt and freshly ground black pepper

2 large heads escarole, coarsely chopped

12 Candied Tomatoes (page 174)

citrus pesto–encrusted fish

1 lemon

1 lime

4 tablespoons extra virgin olive oil

4 garlic cloves

¼ cup finely chopped flat-leaf parsley

¼ cup finely chopped fresh basil

1 large egg

Sea salt and freshly ground black pepper

Two 6-ounce fresh sea bass fillets

1 cup dry white wine (use chicken stock for Detox)

2 tablespoons (¼ stick) unsalted butter

Grate the zests of the lemon and the lime, being careful not to grate the bitter white pith. When finished, squeeze the lemon and lime juice into a bowl and set aside. Place the grated zest, 2 tablespoons of the olive oil, the garlic, parsley, and basil into a food processor. Blend until all the ingredients are finely chopped and well combined. You may need to scrape down the sides. (If you do not have a food processor, chop all the ingredients until very fine and combine.) Pour the mixture onto a plate and set aside.

Place the egg in a shallow bowl and lightly beat. Add salt and pepper. Dip the fish into the egg, then lay the fillets on the parsley mixture to coat. Turn over and coat the other side.

Place a skillet over medium-high heat. Add the remaining 2 tablespoons of olive oil, then the fish, and sauté about 4 minutes per side. Remove the fish and set aside to keep warm.

Add the wine to the hot skillet and turn the heat up to high. Let the wine cook off for a couple of minutes, scraping the browned bits off the bottom of the pan to release the flavors. Add the lemon and lime juice. When the sauce has reduced by half, season with salt and pepper. Turn off the heat and add the butter, 1 tablespoon at a time, swirling until melted.

Serve the fish immediately, with the sauce poured over the top.   SERVES 2

pan-fried petrale sole with lemon butter and caper sauce

PROTEIN, HEALTHY FATS, VEGETABLES

DETOX, LEVEL 1, LEVEL 2

Season both sides of the fish with salt and pepper.

Heat a frying pan on medium-high heat. Add the olive oil to cover the bottom of the pan. When oil is hot, add the fish. Cook 2 to 3 minutes on each side, until fish is brown and crispy. Turn the fish over with a spatula and cook another 2 to 3 minutes on the other side.

Pour the lemon juice over the fish and remove from pan. Set aside. Add the butter and capers to the hot pan. Swirl the butter until melted, scraping any browned bits off the bottom of the pan. Spoon the butter sauce and capers over the fish and serve immediately with lemon wedges. SERVES 2

12 ounces petrale sole or Dover sole fillets

Sea salt and freshly ground black pepper

3 tablespoons olive oil

Juice from 1 lemon

3 tablespoons unsalted butter

1 tablespoon capers

Lemon wedges, for garnish

pan-roasted sole with thyme butter sauce

THYME BUTTER SAUCE

1 shallot, thinly sliced

3 sprigs fresh thyme

5 black peppercorns

1 cup white wine (use chicken stock for Detox)

4 tablespoons ($^1/_2$ stick) unsalted butter

1 tablespoon chopped fresh thyme leaves

SOLE

12 ounces petrale sole or Dover sole fillets

Sea salt and freshly ground black pepper

3 tablespoons olive oil

For the sauce: In a medium saucepan over medium heat, add the shallot, thyme sprigs, peppercorns, and wine. Cook until reduced by three-fourths, then lower the heat and add the butter. Whisk until melted. Strain through a sieve, then add the chopped thyme.

For the sole: Season the fish with salt and pepper. In a medium sauté pan over high heat, add the oil, then add the fish and cook for 2 to 3 minutes on each side, until golden brown. Remove from the heat and place onto plates. Spoon the sauce over the top. Serve immediately. SERVES 2

grilled tuna with lemon-thyme aïoli

PROTEIN, HEALTHY FATS, VEGETABLES

DETOX, LEVEL 1, LEVEL 2

Heat the grill to high.

Drizzle the olive oil over the tuna. Season with salt, pepper, and lemon zest. Grill for 2 minutes per side for medium-rare tuna. To cook through, allow 3 minutes per side.

Place the fish on serving plates. Drizzle with the aïoli and garnish with a fresh sprig of thyme. Serve immediately.   SERVES 2

Olive oil

Two 6-ounce tuna steaks, 1¹/₂ inches thick

Sea salt and freshly ground black pepper

Zest from 1 lemon

1¹/₂ cups Lemon-Thyme Aïoli (recipe follows)

2 sprigs fresh thyme, for garnish

lemon-thyme aïoli

PROTEIN, HEALTHY FATS, VEGETABLES

DETOX, LEVEL 1, LEVEL 2

1 large egg

1 large egg yolk

1 tablespoon Dijon mustard

1 garlic clove, minced

Juice and zest from ¹/₂ lemon

1 tablespoon chopped fresh thyme, or 1 teaspoon dried

Sea salt and freshly ground black pepper

1¹/₂ cups light olive oil

Place all the ingredients, except the oil, into a blender or food processor. Blend until smooth. With the machine running, add the oil in a slow stream until the aïoli becomes emulsified. Serve immediately or store in an airtight container for 2 to 3 days.   MAKES 1¹/₂ CUPS

grilled yellowfin tuna with tomato, fennel, and citrus zest

PROTEIN, HEALTHY FATS, VEGETABLES

DETOX, LEVEL 1, LEVEL 2

1 tablespoon olive oil

$^1/_2$ cup chopped onion

1 fennel bulb, trimmed and sliced (reserve green tops for garnish)

2 garlic cloves, pressed

One 4$^1/_2$-ounce can plum tomatoes with juice

$^1/_2$ teaspoon fennel seeds

3 strips lemon zest

3 strips orange zest

Sea salt and freshly ground black pepper

Four 6-ounce yellowfin tuna (ahi) steaks

4 thin lemon slices, for garnish

Heat a medium skillet over high heat. Add the olive oil, then the onion and fennel. Sauté until the onion is translucent, about 3 minutes. Add the garlic and sauté an additional minute. Add the tomatoes with their juice, the fennel seeds, and the lemon and orange zests. Bring to a boil, then lower the heat and simmer for 15 minutes. Add salt and pepper to taste. Set sauce aside.

Preheat a grill to medium high. Season the tuna steaks with salt and pepper. Grill the fish until barely cooked through—2 to 3 minutes on each side, depending on the thickness of the steaks.

Arrange the steaks on a platter and surround with the sauce. Garnish with the fennel tops and a lemon slice on each tuna steak.   SERVES 4

cilantro-lime grilled tuna

PROTEIN, HEALTHY FATS, VEGETABLES

DETOX, LEVEL 1, LEVEL 2

$^1/_3$ cup fresh lime juice (about 5 limes)

$^2/_3$ cup olive oil

$^1/_4$ cup chopped fresh cilantro

5 garlic cloves, chopped

$^1/_4$ teaspoon sea salt

$^1/_4$ teaspoon freshly ground black pepper

Four 4-ounce tuna steaks, $^1/_2$ inch thick

Place the lime juice, olive oil, cilantro, garlic, salt, and pepper in a bowl. Whisk until the mixture emulsifies and becomes thick. Place the tuna steaks in a large glass or other nonreactive bowl. Pour the marinade into the bowl. Cover and refrigerate for 1 hour.

Heat the grill to medium high. Remove the tuna from the marinade. Grill for 2 to 3 minutes per side, or until tuna is cooked to preferred doneness.   SERVES 4

roasted trout with lemon-sage mayonnaise

PROTEIN, HEALTHY FATS, VEGETABLES

DETOX, LEVEL 1, LEVEL 2

Preheat the oven to 450°F.

Open each trout and season with some lemon juice, salt, pepper, and 4 sage leaves. Close the fish and rub olive oil and additional lemon juice on the exterior. Place trout in a roasting pan and bake for 15 to 20 minutes. Serve garnished with additional lemon wedges, fresh sage leaves, and a drizzle of Lemon-Sage Mayonnaise.   SERVES 4

2 whole trout (1 pound each), cleaned and boned

Juice from 2 lemons

Sea salt and freshly ground black pepper

8 fresh sage leaves

2 to 3 tablespoons olive oil

8 lemon wedges

Fresh sage leaves

1 cup Lemon-Sage Mayonnaise (recipe follows)

lemon-sage mayonnaise

HEALTHY FATS, VEGETABLES

DETOX, LEVEL 1, LEVEL 2

1 recipe Homemade Mayonnaise (page 148)

1 teaspoon finely chopped fresh sage leaves

Juice from 1 lemon

Freshly ground black pepper

Combine all the ingredients in a bowl. Cover and refrigerate to let the flavors mix. Store in an airtight container in the refrigerator for up to 1 week.   MAKES 1 CUP

grilled halibut with spicy rock shrimp salsa

PROTEIN, HEALTHY FATS, VEGETABLES

DETOX, LEVEL 1, LEVEL 2

12 ounces fresh halibut fillet (or other white flaky fish)

Olive oil

Sea salt and freshly ground black pepper

Zest and juice from 1 lemon

4 fresh basil leaves, or 1 teaspoon dried

1 jalapeño chile, seeded and finely diced (see Note, page 39)

½ red onion, finely diced

½ pound rock shrimp (see Note, page 82)

2 tablespoons finely chopped fresh cilantro

Zest and juice from 1 lime

1 tablespoon julienned fresh mint leaves

1 tomato, seeded and finely diced

Drizzle the halibut with olive oil, then season with salt, pepper, lemon zest, and basil leaves. Set aside to let the flavors infuse.

Place a medium sauté pan on high heat. Add 2 tablespoons of olive oil, the jalapeño, and the red onion. Sauté for about 2 minutes, then add the rock shrimp and cook until they turn pink, about 2 minutes more. Pour the ingredients into a mixing bowl and add the cilantro, lime zest and juice, mint, and tomato. Gently toss to combine with a pinch of sea salt.

Heat the grill to high. When hot, add the fish and cook for about 2 minutes per side. Place onto a serving dish and squeeze fresh lemon juice over the top. Add a little more salt and pepper, then top with a generous portion of rock shrimp salsa. Serve immediately. SERVES 2

pan-roasted halibut with zucchini noodles, candied roma tomatoes, and parsley pesto

PROTEIN, HEALTHY FATS, VEGETABLES

DETOX, LEVEL 1, LEVEL 2

Prepare the zucchini in strips and set aside uncooked.

Drizzle the olive oil over the halibut to coat. Season liberally with salt and pepper. Heat a large sauté pan on medium high. Add about 2 tablespoons olive oil and the halibut fillets to fit comfortably in the pan. Sear for 2 minutes per side, or until just cooked through.

Remove the fish from the pan and set aside to keep warm. Return the pan to medium heat and add the zucchini noodles. Season with salt and pepper and sauté for about 30 seconds, until just warmed through.

Place the fish on individual dishes along with zucchini noodles and 3 candied tomatoes per plate. Top the fish with a generous spoonful of pesto and serve immediately.   SERVES 4

1 recipe Zucchini
   Noodles (page 177)

Olive oil

Four 6-ounce halibut
   fillets (or other white
   flaky fish)

Sea salt and freshly
   ground black pepper

12 Candied Tomatoes
   (page 174), made
   with Roma (plum)
   tomatoes

1 cup Parsley Pesto
   (page 150)

herb-crusted halibut steaks with tomato basil sauce

PROTEIN, HEALTHY FATS, VEGETABLES

DETOX, LEVEL 1, LEVEL 2

HALIBUT

Two 6-ounce halibut
  steaks

Sea salt and freshly
  ground black pepper

2 tablespoons finely
  chopped flat-leaf
  parsley

2 tablespoons finely
  chopped fresh basil

1 tablespoon olive oil

TOMATO BASIL SAUCE

1 cup dry white wine
  (use chicken stock
  for Detox)

1 cup chopped tomato

2 tablespoons fresh
  basil leaves,
  julienned

1 tablespoon unsalted
  butter

For the halibut: Rinse the steaks and pat dry. Season both sides of the fish with salt and pepper. Combine the parsley and chopped basil in a small bowl. Make an herb crust on the halibut steaks by pressing the herbs onto both sides of the flesh.

Heat a large skillet over medium-high heat. Add the olive oil, then the fish, and cook for about 3 minutes on each side. Remove the fish and set aside to keep warm.

For the sauce: Add the wine to the hot pan, scraping the browned bits off the bottom of the pan to release the flavor. When the wine has reduced by about one-third, add the tomato and basil, and stir until just heated through. Turn off the heat and add the butter, swirling until combined.

Serve the halibut steaks with the sauce poured over the top.   SERVES 2

ginger scallion grilled mahimahi

PROTEIN, VEGETABLES

DETOX, LEVEL 1, LEVEL 2

1 cup soy sauce

2 teaspoons grated
  fresh ginger

3 garlic cloves, minced

2 scallions, finely
  chopped, plus
  6 whole scallions

Juice of 1 lime

2 mahimahi steaks
  or your favorite fish

Combine the soy sauce, ginger, garlic, chopped scallions, and lime juice in a glass or other nonreactive bowl.

Place the mahimahi in the marinade, cover, and marinate for at least 10 minutes, or in the refrigerator for up to several hours.

Heat the grill to medium high. Remove the fish from the bowl, reserving the marinade. Place the fish and whole scallions on the grill. Grill for 3 minutes per side. Brush the scallions with the marinade, turning as necessary. Serve immediately.   SERVES 2

crispy fried catfish with ginger chips

PROTEIN, HEALTHY FATS, VEGETABLES

DETOX, LEVEL 1, LEVEL 2

One 24-ounce bottle
grapeseed oil

1 large piece fresh
ginger

4 garlic cloves

2 bunches fresh cilantro

2 bunches scallions

Sea salt

Ground white pepper

Four 6-ounce catfish
fillets

Soy sauce

1 lime, quartered

1½ cups Green
Goddess Dressing
(page 146)

Heat the oil in a large frying pan on medium-high heat until it reaches about 350°F.

Peel the ginger, then thinly slice the root on an angle. (You should have about 20 slices.) Peel the garlic and thinly slice on an angle. Wash the cilantro and trim the ends. Wash the scallions and trim the ends. To feather the ends of the scallions, lay each one on the chopping block and slice lengthwise, starting from the light green part down through to the white end. Then turn the scallions and slice again, creating a feathered end.

Begin the frying process with the ginger. Fry the ginger slices until golden brown, about 4 minutes; drain on paper towels. Add the garlic and fry for about 2 minutes; drain on paper towels. Add the cilantro and fry for 2 to 3 minutes; drain on paper towels. Add the scallions and fry for 3 to 4 minutes; drain on paper towels. Salt each item to taste.

Sprinkle a little salt and white pepper on the catfish fillets. Add the catfish to the oil and fry for 2 to 3 minutes, then flip and fry another 2 minutes. Drain on paper towels.

To serve, place a catfish fillet on each plate with a pile of ginger chips, fried garlic, fried cilantro, and fried scallions. Serve with soy sauce, a slice of lime, and a dollop of dressing. SERVES 4

grilled ginger shrimp on skewers

PROTEIN, HEALTHY FATS, VEGETABLES

DETOX, LEVEL 1, LEVEL 2

60 large raw shrimp (fresh or flash-frozen), peeled and deveined

One 4-inch piece fresh ginger, peeled and thinly sliced

2 bunches scallions, chopped into 5-inch pieces

20 garlic cloves, peeled and sliced

2 cups coconut oil

1/2 cup soy sauce

1 teaspoon hot chili oil

2 tablespoons toasted sesame oil

Freshly ground black pepper

12 wooden skewers, soaked in water

Place the shrimp in a large glass or other nonreactive bowl with all the other ingredients and let marinate for at least 2 hours in a cool place.

Prepare the grill by setting to medium high.

Shortly before grilling, thread the shrimp on the bamboo skewers (about 5 shrimp per skewer). Remove the scallions from the marinade and set them aside.

Heat a small frying pan on medium heat. Spoon out all the garlic and ginger slices and a ladleful of the oil in which the shrimp has been marinating, and fry the garlic and ginger for 2 to 3 minutes, or until golden brown and crispy. Set aside.

Place the skewers on the hot grill and cook quickly, about 2 minutes per side. On the same grill, place the marinated scallions and grill until crispy, about 2 minutes. At the last minute, carefully spoon some marinade over the shrimp; use caution as it causes flames to shoot up.

Serve two skewers per person with a spoonful of the fried ginger and garlic, and a couple of grilled scallions.   SERVES 6

pan-fried garlic lemon shrimp with zucchini pesto noodles and arugula

PROTEIN, HEALTHY FATS, VEGETABLES

DETOX, LEVEL 1, LEVEL 2

Place the shrimp in a large bowl. Coat the shrimp with 1 cup olive oil, garlic, lemon juice (reserve some to drizzle on the arugula), parsley, and pepper. Gently toss to distribute flavor. Marinate for at least 2 hours in a cool place. Stir occasionally to marinate evenly.

Toss the cooked zucchini noodles in the pesto. Arrange the noodles on individual dinner plates. Arrange a few arugula leaves around the edge and drizzle with a little extra virgin olive oil, lemon juice, salt, and pepper. Set these plates aside while you prepare the shrimp.

Heat a large frying pan, then ladle as many shrimp as will fit flat, along with a few tablespoons of the marinade, into the hot frying pan. Using a slotted spoon, gather up all the garlic and parsley and include it with the cooking shrimp. Cook the shrimp quickly, 2 to 3 minutes on each side, and then remove from heat.

Season the shrimp with salt. Place the shrimp in the middle of the noodles with a spoonful of the golden brown garlic. Garnish with lemon wedges. SERVES 4 TO 6

60 large raw shrimp (fresh or flash-frozen), peeled and deveined

1 cup olive oil

14 garlic cloves, very thinly sliced

Juice from 3 or 4 lemons

1 bunch flat-leaf parsley, stems removed and leaves coarsely chopped

Freshly ground black pepper

1 recipe Zucchini Noodles (page 177)

1/2 cup Basil-Parsley Pesto (page 150)

8 ounces arugula leaves or baby spinach leaves

Extra virgin olive oil

Sea salt

Lemon wedges, for garnish

scallop skewers

2 tablespoons fresh
lemon juice (about
1 lemon)

1/3 cup fresh lime juice
(about 5 limes)

3 garlic cloves,
chopped

1/2 cup extra virgin olive
oil

1/2 teaspoon sea salt

1/4 teaspoon freshly
ground black pepper

1 pound large scallops

1 large red bell pepper,
cut into 1-inch pieces

1 large onion, quartered
and cut into 1-inch
pieces

1/2 pound medium-size
button mushrooms
(about 15)

Chopped fresh chives,
for garnish

12 wooden skewers,
soaked in water

To make the marinade, mix together the lemon juice, lime juice, garlic, oil, salt, and pepper in a medium bowl. Whisk until smooth and
slightly emulsified. Add the scallops and toss to coat with the marinade. Cover and refrigerate for 1 hour.

To make the skewers, alternate red peppers, onions, mushrooms,
and scallops on 12-inch wooden or metal skewers. Lay the skewers in a
shallow pan. Pour the marinade over the scallops and vegetables.

Preheat a grill. Grill the skewers for 5 to 6 minutes per side, or until
cooked through. Sprinkle with chopped chives before serving.

MAKES 5 SKEWERS

clam bake! mussel bake! crab bake! lobster bake!

PROTEIN, HEALTHY FATS

DETOX, LEVEL 1, LEVEL 2

Clams

Mussels

Lobsters

Crabs, frozen or fresh

Cider vinegar

Old Bay crab boil

Melted unsalted butter, for serving

Lemon wedges

Big stockpot with cover

Steam basket insert (that fits inside the big pot)

To cook clams and mussels, first rinse them in cold water to remove sand and dirt. When these mollusks are fresh, they are still alive. The shells will close automatically when they feel the cold water. If any shells are cracked, broken, or remain open, discard them.

Fill the large pot with 2 to 3 inches of water and layer the clams or mussels in the steam basket insert. Cover. Bring the water to a boil on high heat and occasionally shake the pan. It takes between 5 and 10 minutes to completely steam the mussels or clams. Peek in the pot and remove clams or mussels from heat when their shells are wide open. That means they are cooked.

To steam live lobsters, use the same method as above, allowing about 15 minutes for a 1½-pound lobster. Fresh lobsters will change color from their natural speckled brown tones to a bright red. Increase the cooking time 2 to 3 minutes for every additional ¼ pound.

Many crabs today are precooked and then frozen. To refresh frozen crabs, place them in a pot of boiling water for 1 to 2 minutes and drain. To steam live crabs, you will also need a large pot with a steamer insert. Add equal parts water to cider vinegar and fill the pot just slightly above the bottom of the insert. Layer the crabs with a sprinkling of Old Bay crab boil. Cover the pot. Bring water and vinegar to a boil and steam crabs until they turn bright pink and their legs can be easily pulled from their sockets.

Serve with small bowls of melted butter and lemon wedges.

seafood stew with red pepper rouille

2 tablespoons olive oil

1 onion, thinly sliced

1 fennel bulb, trimmed and thinly sliced

2 garlic cloves, smashed

10 to 12 saffron threads

1 1/2 cups dry white wine (omit for Detox)

8 cups chicken stock or broth, preferably homemade (pages 30–32)

1 tablespoon sea salt

Freshly ground black pepper

12 hard shell clams, preferably littleneck, well scrubbed

16 mussels, well scrubbed

1/2 pound bay scallops

1/2 pound rock shrimp (see Note, page 82), or peeled and deveined shrimp

8 crab legs (optional), scrubbed

1 medium tomato, seeds removed and diced

8 tablespoons (1 stick) unsalted butter, cut into 8 pieces

Juice from 1 lemon

3/4 cup Red Pepper Rouille (page 152)

Place a large stockpot on medium heat. Add the olive oil, onion, fennel, and garlic. Cook for 10 to 15 minutes, until the vegetables are soft. Add the saffron threads and wine, and continue cooking until reduced by half. Add the stock, salt, and a few turns of freshly ground black pepper. Cook slowly over medium heat for another 20 to 30 minutes to let the flavors combine.

Add all the seafood (if the clams are particularly large, add them 3 minutes before the other seafood since they will take longer to open). Add the tomato, cover, and cook for about 5 minutes. Remove the lid and check on the seafood. The shellfish should be opened and the shrimp just cooked through. Discard any unopened shells. Add the butter and swirl to dissolve. Drizzle with lemon juice and serve in large bowls. Garnish with the red pepper rouille. SERVES 4

FOR LEVEL 2 Serve with 2 slices of toasted whole wheat bread with more red pepper rouille.

beef, pork, and lamb

succulent selections

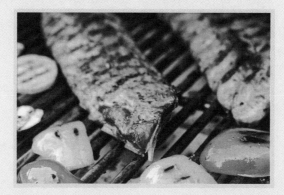

I love the freedom we have with the Sexy Forever plan to enjoy meat. These dishes make for exciting, flavorful meals. It's hard to feel deprived when you can dine on grilled steaks, slow-cooked stews, tender chops, or beautiful roasts. As with most things in life, it's about quality and balance.

I choose grass-fed, pasture-raised, and organic meats whenever possible. And you can taste the difference. Many of these meats are lean, but even if they have a high fat content, those of us on the Sexy Forever plan don't overdo it on portions, as these real foods are filling and satisfy with essential protein. I do not shy away from meat.

When Alan and I were in Tuscany, a wonderful Italian housewife cooked for us and gave me the inspiration for Pan-Fried New York Steaks with Fried Elephant Garlic (page 267). Garnished with fried rosemary and whole red chiles, it takes only about 15 minutes to prepare and it's a "Wow!" In the slow-roasted category, my Twelve-Hour Roast Pork (page 302) shreds into succulent pieces, making an excellent choice for feeding a large crowd. Warning: they won't go home until it's gone! And the Grilled Butterflied

Leg of Lamb (page 285) makes your Easter or Passover holiday something very special. Plus it's surprisingly easy . . . like so many of the recipes in this book.

I also love the summer months for grilling meats outdoors. Meats take to marinades beautifully, and a quick flash on the grill adds an extra bit of character as the meat and marinade sear over the hot fire. Carne Asada (page 272), made with a skirt steak, is a thin cut that cooks in a couple of minutes per side. It's fabulous with Pico de Gallo (page 273). And try my Baby Back Pork Ribs (page 305) for a savory version—something a little different from your regular barbecue sauce.

Go ahead. Take a bite.

christmas standing rib roast

PROTEINS, HEALTHY FATS, VEGETABLES

DETOX, LEVEL 1, LEVEL 2

Preheat the oven to 450°F.

Preheat a large sauté pan over high heat. Add the olive oil. Season the meat heavily with salt and pepper, then carefully sear it on all sides until it forms a dark crust (but not burned), about 3 minutes per side. Make sure all sides are evenly browned. (Use tongs for easier handling.)

Remove the meat from the sauté pan and place into a roasting pan bone side down. Using the string as an anchor, stick the stems of rosemary and thyme under the string so they are secure. Attach the garlic cloves in the same manner. Place the roasting pan into the oven and roast for 30 minutes. Reduce the oven temperature to 350°F. Continue cooking for 1 hour more, or until a meat thermometer registers 125° to 130°F for medium rare, 140°F for medium. Remove the roast from the pan and let it rest for at least 20 minutes before carving.

Meanwhile, pour the fat out of the roasting pan and place the pan over medium heat. Add the shallots and allow them to caramelize while scraping browned bits from the bottom of the pan. Add the wine and reduce by half. Add the veal demi-glace and stock. Simmer for 2 to 3 minutes. Stir in the butter and season with salt and pepper. Carve the meat and serve with a spoonful of sauce. SERVES 6

2 tablespoons olive oil

One 7- to 8-pound standing rib roast (ask butcher to tie it but leave the bone attached)

Sea salt and freshly ground black pepper

1 bunch fresh rosemary

1 bunch fresh thyme

1 head garlic, cloves separated

2 shallots, finely diced

1 cup good red wine (use stock for Detox)

1 cup veal demi-glace (see Note)

$\frac{1}{2}$ cup beef stock, preferably homemade (page 34)

2 tablespoons ($\frac{1}{4}$ stick) unsalted butter

NOTE The demi-glace is a special treat and well worth buying (or ordering online) from your local gourmet store. If you can't find it, use additional stock or wine in its place.

beef tournedos in burgundy sauce

BAKED GARLIC

1 head garlic

Olive oil

Fresh or dried thyme

TOURNEDOS

1 pound beef tenderloin, cut into 4 fillets (ask your butcher to do this for you)

Sea salt and freshly ground black pepper

2 tablespoons olive oil

1 shallot, minced

1 cup beef stock, preferably homemade (page 34)

¼ cup burgundy wine (use stock for Detox)

2 tablespoons tomato puree

2 tablespoons (¼ stick) unsalted butter

Chopped flat-leaf parsley

For the baked garlic: Preheat the oven to 350°F. Slice the top off the head of garlic, exposing the cluster of cloves. Brush with a touch of olive oil and sprinkle with thyme. Place in a shallow baking dish and bake for 45 minutes, or until golden brown and bubbly. Remove from the heat and set aside.

For the tournedos: Squeeze about 8 of the baked garlic cloves out of their skins; save the rest for another use. Rub the filets all over with the roasted garlic. Season with salt and pepper. Heat a skillet over medium-high heat. Add the olive oil and as many of the filets as will fit into the pan. Brown for 2 to 3 minutes per side. Remove from the pan and keep warm. Repeat until all the filets are browned, adding more oil as necessary.

When all the meat is cooked, add the shallot and cook until tender, about 3 minutes. Add the stock and wine. Turn the heat up to high, scraping the browned bits from the bottom of the pan to release the flavor. Let the sauce reduce by half. Add the tomato puree, stirring until heated through. Turn off the heat and add the butter, 1 tablespoon at a time, until well combined.

Place the filets on a plate and top with the sauce. Garnish with the parsley. SERVES 4

filet mignon au poivre

PROTEIN, HEALTHY FATS, VEGETABLES

DETOX, LEVEL 1, LEVEL 2

Pat the steaks dry with a paper towel and sprinkle with salt. Bring to room temperature.

Place the white and black peppercorns on a cutting board and crack them with a heavy pan. Rub the steaks on both sides with salt and the cracked pepper, pushing the peppercorn bits into the meat.

In a large skillet, heat 1 tablespoon of the butter and the olive oil over medium-high heat. Place the steaks in the pan and cook for 3 to 4 minutes per side for medium rare, 5 to 6 minutes for medium. Remove the steaks to a platter. Remove the bacon and discard.

Pour off any excess fat from the skillet and return to the heat. Add the port wine and bring to a boil while scraping the browned bits from the bottom of the pan. Add the stock and continue cooking over medium-high heat, reducing the sauce until it is rich and syrupy. Lower the heat and blend in the cream, if desired. Remove from the heat and add the remaining tablespoon of butter to the sauce, stirring until melted. Serve each filet with a generous spoonful of sauce. SERVES 4

Four 6-ounce filet
    mignon steaks,
    wrapped with bacon

Sea salt

1 tablespoon white
    peppercorns

1 tablespoon black
    peppercorns

2 tablespoons (¼ stick)
    unsalted butter

1 tablespoon olive oil

2 tablespoons port
    wine (use stock for
    Detox)

2 tablespoons beef
    stock, preferably
    homamde (page 34)

¼ cup heavy cream
    (optional)

peppered filet of beef with bourbon sauce

PROTEIN, HEALTHY FATS, VEGETABLES

LEVEL 1, LEVEL 2

Four 5- to 6-ounce filet
steaks, trimmed

Sea salt

2 tablespoons black
peppercorns,
crushed

4 tablespoons (½ stick)
unsalted butter

4 slices bacon

3 garlic cloves,
chopped

⅔ cup dry red wine

2 tablespoons bourbon

Season the steaks with salt. Place the peppercorns on a cutting board and crack them with a heavy pan. Sprinkle the steaks with the crushed peppercorns, pressing the pepper into the meat. Set aside.

Heat a medium skillet on high heat. Melt 1 tablespoon of the butter. Add the bacon and cook until crisp. Drain the bacon on paper towels. Cool, then crumble. Reserve.

Using the same skillet, turn the heat to high and add the steaks. For rare, cook 1½ to 2 minutes on each side; for medium-rare, 2½ to 3 minutes on each side. Add more time for well done. Remove steaks to a platter and cover loosely to keep warm.

Add another tablespoon of butter to the skillet, put over medium heat, and brown the chopped garlic for 1 to 2 minutes. Add the wine and bring to a boil. Stir constantly, loosening the browned bits on the bottom of the pan. Simmer the liquid until reduced by half. Turn off heat, whisk in the remaining 2 tablespoons butter, and add the bourbon. Place the steaks on four serving plates. Add the bacon pieces to the sauce, and drizzle the sauce over the meat. SERVES 4

pan-roasted rib-eye with sweet onion and sautéed spinach

PROTEIN, HEALTHY FATS, VEGETABLES

DETOX, LEVEL 1, LEVEL 2

1 red onion

1 tablespoon balsamic vinegar

Extra virgin olive oil

Sea salt and freshly ground black pepper

2 slices bacon

1 bunch fresh thyme, or 3 teaspoons dried

A 1-pound rib-eye steak, 2 inches thick, or a Spencer or New York strip steak

2 garlic cloves, minced

12 ounces baby spinach leaves

Juice from 1 lemon

Preheat the oven to 350°F.

Peel the red onion and slice it through the middle into thirds. Stack back together and drizzle with the balsamic vinegar, about 1 tablespoon olive oil, salt, and pepper. Wrap the slices of bacon around the onion and tuck 1 sprig of fresh thyme (or 1 teaspoon dried) under the bacon. Place in a shallow baking dish. Roast for about 1 hour, or until soft. Remove the bacon, coarsely chop, and reserve to cook with the spinach. Coarsely chop the onion and set aside.

Preheat the oven to 500°F.

Drizzle olive oil over the steak to coat well. Season with salt, pepper, the remaining sprigs of thyme, and 1 clove of the minced garlic. Heat an ovenproof sauté pan on high heat. Add about 2 tablespoons olive oil. Sear the steak for about 2½ minutes on each side, then place the sauté pan into the oven. Roast for 2 minutes, turn the steak over, and continue roasting for another 2 minutes. Remove the steak from the pan, being extremely cautious of the hot handle. Pour off any fat and add the chopped roasted onion, warming on medium heat while scraping browned bits off the bottom of the pan.

Heat a separate sauté pan over medium-high heat. Add 1 tablespoon of olive oil, the reserved bacon, and the remaining minced garlic. Sauté for about 2 minutes. Add the spinach leaves and lemon juice, and toss until just wilted, about 3 minutes.

Slice the steak on the diagonal and divide between two plates. Place some sautéed spinach next to each steak. Then spoon the onion atop the steak and serve immediately. SERVES 2

porterhouse steak

¼ cup extra virgin olive oil

12 garlic cloves, thinly sliced

4 sprigs fresh rosemary

4 sprigs fresh oregano

4 sprigs fresh thyme

One 28-ounce porterhouse steak, at room temperature

Sea salt and freshly ground black pepper

Preheat the broiler.

Heat a skillet over medium heat. Add the olive oil. When the oil is hot, add the garlic, rosemary, oregano, and thyme. Cook until the garlic is golden, 1 to 2 minutes. Set aside to cool.

Season the steak liberally with salt and pepper. Place on a broiling pan and set under the broiler for 4 to 5 minutes per side for medium rare to medium. Transfer to a large plate. Pour the garlic, herbs, and oil over the steak. Let it rest about 10 minutes. Then slice on the diagonal and serve each plate with some of the garlic and herbs. SERVES 4

grilled steaks provençal

PROTEIN, HEALTHY FATS, VEGETABLES

DETOX, LEVEL 1, LEVEL 2

Heat a grill to medium high.

Trim the excess fat from the steak and let sit at room temperature
for 10 minutes. Rub the steak on both sides with 4 tablespoons of olive
oil and salt and pepper.

Place a skillet with the remaining 4 tablespoons oil over medium-
high heat. Add the onions and peppers and cook until golden brown,
20 to 30 minutes. Season with salt and pepper. Add the butter and toss
well.

Place the steak on the hot grill. Cook 6 to 7 minutes per side for
medium.

To serve, place a pile of peppers and onions on each plate. Remove
the steak from the grill. Let the meat rest for 10 minutes. Slice the steak
against the grain and place on top of the peppers and onions. Garnish
each plate with a lemon wedge to squeeze over the steak.   SERVES 4

One 28-ounce
   porterhouse steak

8 tablespoons olive oil

Sea salt and coarsely
   ground black pepper

2 sweet onions (Vidalia
   or Maui), thinly
   sliced

2 medium red bell
   peppers, julienned

2 medium yellow bell
   peppers, julienned

1 tablespoon unsalted
   butter

1 lemon, quartered

grilled pepper steak with herb butter

1 New York strip steak
(2 pounds), trimmed
of fat

3 tablespoons olive oil

4 tablespoons black
peppercorns

4 garlic cloves, minced

Sea salt to taste

2 tablespoons (¼ stick)
unsalted butter

1 teaspoon finely
chopped fresh basil

1 teaspoon finely
chopped fresh
thyme

Heat a grill to high. Pierce the steak all over with a fork to let the oil penetrate. Rub with olive oil.

Crack the peppercorns on a cutting board with a heavy pan. Combine with the garlic and salt to make a paste. Cover both sides of the steak with the mixture.

Grill the steak for 4 to 5 minutes per side for medium rare, 6 to 7 minutes per side for medium. Remove from heat and let rest for 10 minutes.

Melt the butter in a small saucepan and add the herbs. Slice the steak on the diagonal and drizzle with the herb butter. SERVES 2 OR 3

pan-fried new york steaks with fried elephant garlic

PROTEIN, HEALTHY FATS, VEGETABLES

DETOX, LEVEL 1, LEVEL 2

2 tablespoons black peppercorns

Two 2¼-inch-thick New York steaks, flattened

⅓ cup extra virgin olive oil

4 elephant garlic cloves (or 8 regular cloves), thinly sliced

2 teaspoons sea salt

1 tablespoon fresh rosemary leaves, or 1 teaspoon dried

4 fresh rosemary sprigs

4 whole dried red chiles

Crack the peppercorns on a cutting board with a heavy pan. Brush the steaks with a little olive oil. Rub one of the sliced garlic cloves over both sides of the meat. Combine the salt, cracked peppercorns, and rosemary leaves. Season the steaks on both sides with this mixture.

Heat a skillet with the remaining olive oil over medium heat. When the oil is hot, add the rest of the garlic and sauté until golden brown, about 5 minutes. Remove the garlic and set aside. Add the rosemary sprigs, pressing them flat against the bottom of the skillet with a spatula until crispy, about 2 minutes on each side. Remove and set aside. Add the chiles and toss in the hot oil for 30 seconds. Remove and set aside.

Fry the steaks in the infused hot oil, adding more oil if necessary, 2 to 3 minutes on each side. Top the steaks with the garlic, rosemary sprigs, and chiles. Serve immediately. SERVES 2

½ cup port wine

1 cup olive oil

2 garlic cloves, minced

2 tablespoons dry mustard

2 teaspoons soy sauce

1 teaspoon fresh lemon juice

Sea salt and freshly ground black pepper

Dash of hot pepper sauce

Dash of Worcestershire sauce (see Note, page 45)

4 Milanese beef cutlets (thinly pounded slices of sirloin steak)

MUSHROOMS AND ONIONS

6 tablespoons extra virgin olive oil

3 large onions, sliced

1 pound white mushrooms

2 teaspoons dried thyme

½ cup port wine

1 cup beef stock, preferably homemade (page 34)

Sea salt and freshly ground black pepper

2 tablespoons (¼ stick) unsalted butter

TO FINISH

2 cups port wine

2 tablespoons (¼ stick) unsalted butter

milanese beef with sautéed onions and mushrooms in a port wine sauce

PROTEIN, HEALTHY FATS, VEGETABLES

LEVEL 1, LEVEL 2

For the meat: Combine all the ingredients except the beef in a glass or other nonreactive bowl. Add the steaks and marinate 6 to 24 hours, turning the steaks after half the time has passed.

For the mushrooms and onions: Heat a large skillet over medium heat. Add 3 tablespoons of olive oil. Add the onions and sauté until they become golden brown and begin to caramelize, about 10 minutes. Add the mushrooms. Continue stirring and add the remaining 3 table-spoons oil and the thyme. As they cook, the mushrooms will release all of their liquid. Continue cooking them down until the liquid has cooked off, approximately 15 minutes. At this point they will begin to get brown and crusty on the edges.

Turn the heat up to high and add the port and the stock. Stir the mushrooms and wine, scraping the bottom of the pan to release the flavor. Add salt and pepper to taste. Continue to cook over high heat until the liquid is reduced by half. Turn off the heat and add the butter. Stir to combine.

To finish: Let the steaks sit out at room temperature for 15 minutes before cooking. Heat a large skillet over medium-high heat. Remove the steaks from the marinade and place as many as will fit flat in the pan. Cook for 2 minutes on each side. Remove and set aside in a warm place until all the steaks are cooked.

Place the pan over high heat and add the 2 cups port. Scrape the browned bits off the bottom of the pan to release the flavor. When the sauce has reduced by half, turn off the heat and add the butter, 1 tablespoon at a time, swirling until combined.

Serve each steak topped with a pile of mushrooms and the port sauce. SERVES 4

rosemary london broil

PROTEIN, HEALTHY FATS, VEGETABLES

DETOX, LEVEL 1, LEVEL 2

1 teaspoon black peppercorns

2 garlic cloves, pressed

2 tablespoons chopped fresh rosemary

1 tablespoon grated lemon zest

2 tablespoons olive oil

1 cup dry red wine (omit for Detox)

One 2-pound London broil

2 tablespoons (¼ stick) unsalted butter

Crack the peppercorns on a cutting board with a heavy pan.

Place the garlic and rosemary in a large glass or other nonreactive bowl. With a large spoon, mash or press the garlic and rosemary, releasing the flavors. Add the cracked peppercorns and lemon zest, and mash together. Add the oil and half the wine.

Score the meat on the top and bottom with a knife by cutting an *X* into the meat about ⅛ inch thick. Place the meat in the marinade for at least 15 minutes, turning after half the time has expired. (Flavor is best if marinated overnight in the refrigerator.)

Let the meat sit out at room temperature for 15 minutes before cooking. Heat a grill to high.

Remove the meat from the marinade, reserving the marinade, and place on the grill. For medium rare, the meat will take approximately 5 minutes per side for a 1½-inch-thick London broil, 7 minutes per side for medium. Let the meat rest for 10 minutes.

Meanwhile, strain the marinade. Discard the rosemary, peppercorns, and lemon zest. Place the liquid in a skillet over high heat. Let the marinade reduce by about one-third. Add the remaining ½ cup wine. Let the liquid reduce by half, then turn off the heat. Add the butter, 1 tablespoon at a time, and stir until melted.

Thinly slice the London broil on an angle and serve with the sauce. SERVES 4

greek beef kebabs

PROTEIN, HEALTHY FATS, VEGETABLES

DETOX, LEVEL 1, LEVEL 2

1 pound boneless sirloin steak, cut into 2-inch cubes

¼ cup olive oil

1 tablespoon dried oregano

Sea salt and freshly ground black pepper

24 pearl onions, peeled (see Note, page 277)

24 cherry tomatoes, stems removed

3 red or green bell peppers, seeded and chopped into 2-inch squares

24 white mushrooms, stems removed

8 metal skewers or wooden skewers, soaked in water

Place the sirloin cubes, olive oil, oregano, salt, and pepper in a glass or other nonreactive bowl. Marinate meat in the refrigerator at least 1 hour or as long as overnight. Drain and reserve the marinade for basting.

Heat a grill to high. To make the kebabs, skewer the meat and vegetables on 12-inch skewers in a pattern. Thread the next kebab and continue until all ingredients are used.

Over very high heat, lay the kebabs on the grill and cook, basting with leftover marinade, and turning as needed until the meat is done to your liking, about 6 minutes for medium. MAKES 8 KEBABS

beef stroganoff

PROTEIN, HEALTHY FATS, VEGETABLES

DETOX, LEVEL 1, LEVEL 2

Trim any silver skin from the tenderloin, then cut across the width into 1-inch slices. Slightly flatten the slices by pressing with the palm of your hand. Set aside.

Place a medium skillet over medium-high heat, add the butter, and melt. Sauté the mushrooms with the salt and pepper until golden, about 5 minutes. Add the pickles and juice, and cook until the juice evaporates slightly, about 2 minutes. Add the cream and cook until reduced by half.

Meanwhile, season the meat with a little salt and pepper (the sauce will be salty from the pickles). Heat a large skillet over high heat and add the oil. When the oil is hot, sear the meat briefly, 2 minutes per side for medium rare.

Place the spinach on plates, top with the beef, then ladle the warm sauce over the top. SERVES 6

2^1/2 pounds beef tenderloin

1 tablespoon unsalted butter

2^1/2 cups sliced white mushrooms

^{1}/4 teaspoon sea salt, plus more to taste

Freshly ground black pepper

1^1/2 cups julienned dill pickles, with 2 tablespoons pickle juice

2 cups heavy cream

2 tablespoons olive oil

Sautéed Spinach with Garlic, Lemon, and Oil (page 172)

carne asada

2 pounds skirt steak

2 bunches cilantro, roughly chopped

1 onion, roughly chopped

1 tomato, roughly chopped

1 cup fresh lemon juice

1 orange, sliced with peel (omit for Detox)

Sea salt

1 recipe Pico de Gallo (recipe follows)

Sour cream, for garnish

Place the steak in a glass or other nonreactive bowl. Add the cilantro, onion, tomato, lemon juice, orange slices, and salt, making sure the meat is surrounded by the chopped vegetables. Place the bowl in the refrigerator and let marinate overnight (at least 8 hours). Turn the meat once so that the lemon juice marinates both sides equally. Remove the meat from the marinade and discard the marinade.

Heat a grill or broiler. Let the meat sit out at room temperature for about 15 minutes.

Place the meat on the grill or under a broiler for 4 to 5 minutes per side for medium rare, 6 to 7 minutes per side for medium.

Slice on the diagonal into thin strips. Serve immediately with pico de gallo and sour cream.   SERVES 4

NOTE The orange slices create a minor imbalance. You get most of the flavor from the tangy peel. If you are doing well on Level 1, this minor addition should not create a problem.

pico de gallo

VEGETABLES

DETOX, LEVEL 1, LEVEL 2

    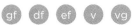

4 ripe medium tomatoes, diced

1/2 medium cucumber, diced

1 bunch cilantro, coarsely chopped

1 red onion, diced

2 serrano chiles, finely chopped, with seeds (see Note, page 39)

1 garlic clove, minced

Juice of 2 limes

Gently combine all the ingredients in a glass or other nonreactive bowl and set aside for the flavors to combine, about 30 minutes. Do not refrigerate or the tomatoes will get mealy. MAKES ABOUT 2 CUPS

beef fajitas

1 pound sirloin steak, cut into 1¹/2-inch strips

2 tablespoons Tex-Mex Seasoning (recipe follows)

2 tablespoons fresh lime juice

3 tablespoons olive oil

1 large onion, sliced

2 red bell peppers, cored and sliced into ¹/4-inch strips

3 garlic cloves, crushed

8 to 10 Egg Crêpes (page 35) or whole wheat tortillas (omit for Detox)

GARNISH
Sour cream

Salsa

Shredded cheese

Chopped fresh cilantro

Lime wedges

Toss together the steak, seasoning, and lime juice in a nonreactive bowl. Set aside.

Heat the oil in a large sauté pan over high heat. Add the onion and cook for 35 minutes. Add the peppers and cook for 5 more minutes. Add the garlic and cook for another minute. Then add the steak and cook for 2 minutes.

Heat the crêpes or tortillas in a warm oven for 5 minutes, or microwave for 1 minute. Place the fajita mixture on the crêpes and serve with the garnishes.   SERVES 8 TO 10

tex-mex seasoning

FREE FOOD
DETOX, LEVEL 1, LEVEL 2

1 tablespoon plus 1 teaspoon cayenne

3 tablespoons dried oregano

3 tablespoons ground cumin

1 tablespoon ground coriander

2 teaspoons freshly ground black pepper

2 teaspoons sea salt

Combine all the ingredients in a jar or resealable container. Shake until blended. Store in an airtight container for up to 6 months.   MAKES ABOUT ¹/2 CUP

beef stir-fry

PROTEIN, HEALTHY FATS, VEGETABLES

DETOX, LEVEL 1, LEVEL 2

Place the sliced beef, garlic, ½ cup of the oil, the lemon juice, and a few grinds of black pepper in a glass or other nonreactive bowl. Set aside and marinate for 20 to 30 minutes.

Heat a wok or large sauté pan over high heat. Add 2 tablespoons oil. Add the broccoli and sauté for 60 to 90 seconds; place the broccoli in a large bowl and set aside. Add the baby bok choy and sauté for 60 to 90 seconds; place the bok choy in the bowl with the broccoli. Add another tablespoon of oil and the mushrooms. Sauté for about 2 minutes, then set aside with the other vegetables. Add the snap peas to the pan (with a little more oil, if necessary) and sauté for 1 minute, then set aside with the other vegetables. Add the bean sprouts to the pan and sauté for 45 seconds, then set aside with the other vegetables.

Remove the beef and garlic from the bowl and place in the hot pan, adding the remaining tablespoon oil. Sauté for about 2½ minutes, until just cooked through. Place the vegetables back into the pan and toss everything together with the soy sauce for about 30 seconds. Serve immediately. For a spicy stir-fry, add a few drops of hot pepper oil or a pinch of red pepper flakes. SERVES 4

One 1¼-pound London broil, sliced into ⅛-inch strips

3 garlic cloves, thinly sliced

About ¾ cup olive oil

Juice from 1 lemon

Freshly ground black pepper

3 cups chopped broccoli florets

3 baby bok choy, julienned

2 cups sliced white mushrooms

1 cup julienned snap peas

1 cup bean sprouts

¼ cup soy sauce

Hot pepper oil or red pepper flakes (optional)

in-a-hurry beef curry

2 tablespoons olive oil

A 1-pound piece top
round or sirloin
steak, sliced into
$^1/_4$-inch-thick pieces

1 medium onion,
chopped

1 red bell pepper,
chopped

One 14-ounce can diced
tomatoes

$^2/_3$ cup mild or hot Thai
curry paste

1 tablespoon All Natural
SomerSweet

$^1/_2$ cup heavy cream

3 cups Cucumber Dill
Dip (recipe follows)

Place a large sauté pan over medium-high heat. When hot, add the olive oil and beef. Sauté for 2 to 3 minutes, until browned. Remove the steak from the pan and set aside. Add the onion and cook for 2 minutes. Add the pepper and cook for another 2 minutes. Stir in the tomatoes, curry paste, All Natural SomerSweet, and cream. Bring to a boil, reduce the heat, and simmer for 10 minutes. Return the steak to the pan and simmer for 5 minutes. Serve hot with cucumber dip on the side to cool the spice.   SERVES 6

cucumber dill dip

4 medium cucumbers, peeled, seeded, and cut into 1-inch pieces

$^2/_3$ cup chopped onion

1 bunch fresh dill, stems removed

$2^1/_4$ cups full-fat sour cream

1 tablespoon plus 1 teaspoon fresh lemon juice

2 teaspoons sea salt

$^1/_4$ teaspoon freshly ground black pepper

Place cucumbers, onion, dill, sour cream, lemon juice, salt, and pepper in the bowl of a food processor. Pulse until mixture is the consistency of salsa. Chill for 1 hour.

MAKES 3 CUPS

beef stew

PROTEIN, HEALTHY FATS, VEGETABLES

DETOX, LEVEL 1, LEVEL 2

Heat a large 6-quart Dutch oven or soup pot over medium-high heat. Melt the butter, then add the bacon and cook until the pieces are brown. Drain on paper towels, then crumble and reserve.

Over high heat, sear the beef in the bacon drippings until light brown, 3 to 4 minutes. Remove and reserve with the bacon. In the same pan, add the chopped onion and cook until translucent, 5 minutes. Add the garlic and cook for 1 minute. Add the celery, celery root, pearl onions, and mushrooms, stirring constantly for about 5 minutes. Add the bay leaf, thyme, stock, wine, and tomato sauce. Bring to a boil. Immediately turn the heat down to a simmer, return the bacon and beef to the pot, and cook, covered, for 20 minutes. Remove the cover and add the green beans. Continue to cook until the meat and vegetables are tender when pierced with a fork, approximately 15 minutes.

SERVES 4 TO 6

NOTE For easy peeling, place the pearl onions in a bowl, cover with boiling water for 60 seconds, squeeze them, and the skin slips right off.

1 tablespoon unsalted butter

4 ounces bacon strips

2 pounds trimmed beef round, cut into 1-inch cubes

1 onion, chopped

2 garlic cloves, chopped

3 celery stalks, chopped

1 medium celery root, chopped

12 pearl onions (see Note)

8 ounces white button or other small mushrooms

1 dried bay leaf

1 teaspoon fresh thyme, or $^{1}/_{2}$ teaspoon dried

2 cups beef stock, preferably homemade (page 34)

2 cups dry red wine (use stock for Detox)

1 cup tomato sauce

1 cup sliced green beans

double-double cheeseburgers

PROTEIN, HEALTHY FATS, VEGETABLES

DETOX, LEVEL 1, LEVEL 2

1½ pounds ground
   sirloin

Sea salt and freshly
   ground black pepper

2 tablespoons olive oil

8 slices American or
   Cheddar cheese

1 head iceberg or
   limestone lettuce,
   leaves washed and
   separated

1 red onion, sliced

1 large tomato, sliced

8 dill pickle slices

8 tablespoons Secret
   Sauce (page 152)

Preheat the broiler.

Form the beef into 8 wide, thin patties. Season liberally with salt and pepper. Heat the olive oil in a large skillet over medium-high heat. Add the patties and cook for 3 minutes per side, or until the meat is cooked through.

Place the burgers on a baking sheet. Top each with a slice of cheese. Place under the broiler until the cheese melts. Remove from the broiler.

Lay 4 large lettuce leaves on a work surface. Top each with 1 burger. Place a slice each of onion and tomato and 2 slices of pickle on top of each. Generously spoon on the sauce. Stack the other 4 burgers to create 4 Double-Doubles.

Top with more sauce, if desired. Add another lettuce leaf on top, then fold lettuce over the burgers. Wrap burgers in paper napkins and serve immediately.   SERVES 4

persian kebabs (middle eastern burgers)

PROTEIN, HEALTHY FATS, VEGETABLES

DETOX, LEVEL 1, LEVEL 2

1 large onion

2 pounds ground beef

2 tablespoons
   Koubideh, Persian
   kebab seasoning
   (see Note)

Grate the onion over a plate to catch all the juices. Combine the hamburger meat with the grated onion and juice. Add the seasoning and mash together with your hands until well combined. Refrigerate 6 to 24 hours. (The longer the meat sits, the better the flavor.)

Heat the grill to medium high.

Form the meat into ¼-pound egg-shaped patties (not completely flattened but slightly dome-shaped). Grill over medium-high heat for 8 to 10 minutes, turning frequently to brown all sides.   SERVES 4 TO 6

NOTE Koubideh is available at Middle Eastern and gourmet markets.

puerto rican picadillo

PROTEIN, HEALTHY FATS, VEGETABLES

DETOX, LEVEL 1, LEVEL 2

2 tablespoons olive oil

2 medium onions, finely chopped

1 large bell pepper, finely chopped

6 plum tomatoes, chopped

Sea salt and freshly ground black pepper

1 teaspoon minced fresh garlic

1 teaspoon ground cumin

1 teaspoon ground coriander

1 pound lean ground beef

1 pound ground pork

3/4 cup balsamic vinegar

2 tablespoons capers, drained

1/2 cup tomato puree

Sour cream, for serving

1 bunch cilantro, chopped, for serving

1 head Boston lettuce (optional)

Heat the olive oil in a large skillet over medium heat. Add the onions and pepper. Cook until brown and tender, 10 to 15 minutes. Then add the tomatoes, salt and pepper to taste, garlic, cumin, and coriander.

Turn the heat up to medium high and add the ground beef and ground pork. Brown the meat, using a wooden spoon to break it into tiny pieces. Add the balsamic vinegar, capers, and tomato puree. Reduce the heat and simmer for at least 1 hour.

Serve in a bowl with a dollop of sour cream and chopped cilantro. Or roll up in a lettuce leaf and eat like a taco. SERVES 8

caroline's meat sauce and zucchini noodles

PROTEIN, HEALTHY FATS, VEGETABLES
DETOX, LEVEL 1, LEVEL 2

For the sauce: Place a large stockpot on medium heat. Add the olive oil and onions. Sauté until the onions are translucent, 7 to 10 minutes. Add the garlic and sauté for 1 to 2 minutes longer. Add the ground beef and sauté until brown, about 7 minutes. Season the meat with about ½ teaspoon salt, ½ teaspoon pepper, and the paprika.

Add all 5 cans of tomatoes, roughly chopping the whole peeled tomatoes, including their juice. Add the remaining 1 tablespoon salt, remaining 2 teaspoons pepper, the basil, bay leaves, cayenne, parsley, oregano, and wine. Stir all ingredients until well combined. Bring to a low boil, then lower the heat and simmer for 1 to 4 hours. (The sauce will be ready after an hour but tastes better the longer you simmer it.)

For the meatballs: Preheat the broiler. Drizzle olive oil on a baking sheet until the sheet is completely coated.

Combine the meat, garlic, parsley, eggs, cheese, Worcestershire sauce, salt, and pepper in a bowl. Use your hands to blend the ingredients. Form the meat into small round balls, about 1 inch in diameter. Place the meatballs on the oiled baking sheet. Broil for about 5 minutes, turning as necessary to cook all sides.

Remove the bay leaves from the sauce. Serve the meatballs atop zucchini noodles and pour sauce over. MAKES ABOUT 4 QUARTS

MEAT SAUCE
3 tablespoons olive oil

2 onions, chopped

1 head garlic, minced

2 pounds ground beef

1 tablespoon plus
   ½ teaspoon sea salt

2½ teaspoons freshly
   ground black pepper

2 teaspoons paprika

Two 28-ounce cans
   tomato sauce

Two 28-ounce cans
   tomato puree

One 28-ounce can
   peeled whole
   tomatoes

2 tablespoons dried
   basil

2 dried bay leaves,
   cracked

½ teaspoon cayenne

6 tablespoons finely
   chopped parsley

½ teaspoon dried
   oregano

1 cup dry red wine (omit
   for Detox)

MEATBALLS
Olive oil

1 pound ground beef

3 garlic cloves, minced

3 tablespoons finely
   chopped parsley

2 large eggs, lightly
   beaten

¼ cup freshly grated
   Parmesan cheese

3 dashes Worcester-
   shire sauce (see
   Note, page 45)

Sea salt and freshly
   ground black pepper

Zucchini Noodles
   (page 177)

braised veal stew with gremolata

1/4 cup olive oil

2 pounds veal stew meat (or beef stew meat)

1 veal shank (or beef shank)

1 onion, medium diced

6 celery stalks, medium diced

2 carrots, medium diced (omit for Level 1)

3 tablespoons tomato paste

1 1/2 cups dry red wine

2 tablespoons veal demi-glace (see Note, page 259)

4 cups chicken stock or broth, or more to cover, preferably homemade (pages 30–32)

2 sprigs fresh thyme, or 1 teaspoon dried

4 sprigs flat-leaf parsley, or 2 teaspoons dried

1/2 head garlic

1/2 cup Gremolata (recipe follows)

Heat a large sauté pan on high heat. Add the olive oil, stew meat, and shank. Sauté until browned on the outside, about 5 minutes. Transfer the meat to a slow cooker (see Note).

Return the sauté pan to the heat and add the onion, celery, and carrots (for Level 2). Cook for 3 to 4 minutes, until slightly browned. Add the tomato paste and stir into the vegetables for 2 to 3 minutes. Add the wine, scraping any browned bits off the bottom of the pan to release the flavor. Cook for about 10 minutes, then pour into the slow cooker.

Add the veal demi-glace, chicken stock, thyme, parsley, and garlic (with skin) to the slow cooker. Cover and cook on low for 8 hours.

Ladle into serving bowls and sprinkle with gremolata.   SERVES 6

NOTE If you don't have a slow cooker, bring the stew to a simmer in a Dutch oven, then cover and cook in a 375°F oven for 2½ hours.

gremolata

1/2 bunch flat-leaf parsley leaves, finely minced

Zest from 1 lemon

1 garlic clove, pressed

1/4 cup extra virgin olive oil

Sea salt and freshly ground black pepper

Place all the ingredients into a bowl and toss to combine. Let the flavors meld for 30 minutes. Store in an airtight container in the refrigerator for up to 1 week.   MAKES 1/2 CUP

veal patties with lemon-caper sauce

PROTEIN, HEALTHY FATS, VEGETABLES

DETOX, LEVEL 1, LEVEL 2

Heat a large sauté pan over high heat. Add the olive oil.

Form the veal into 4 patties and season with salt and pepper. Dip each patty first in the Parmesan cheese and then into the beaten egg. Gently place the patties into the sauté pan, being careful not to splash the oil. Cook on each side until golden brown, about 3 minutes. Transfer to a warm platter and set aside.

Reduce the heat to medium. In the same sauté pan, add the capers, garlic, lemon zest, lemon juice, and wine, carefully scraping any bits from the bottom of the pan. Allow the wine to reduce by half. Add the butter and stir until melted. Pour the sauce over the patties and serve immediately.   SERVES 4

2 tablespoons olive oil

1 pound ground veal (or ground dark-meat turkey)

Sea salt and freshly ground black pepper

1 cup freshly grated Parmesan cheese

2 large eggs, slightly beaten

2 teaspoons drained capers

1 garlic clove, finely minced

Zest and juice from 1 lemon

1/4 cup dry white wine (use chicken stock for Detox)

2 tablespoons (1/4 stick) unsalted butter

roasted leg of lamb

One 7- to 8-pound
whole leg of lamb

8 garlic cloves, halved

2 tablespoons extra
virgin olive oil

2 tablespoons dried
rosemary

2 tablespoons dried
thyme

Sea salt and freshly
ground black pepper

1 cup beef stock,
preferably
homemade
(page 34)

1 cup dry red wine (use
stock for Detox)

2 tablespoons (¹⁄4 stick)
unsalted butter

PROTEIN, HEALTHY FATS, VEGETABLES

DETOX, LEVEL 1, LEVEL 2

Preheat the oven to 350°F.

Using a small paring knife, make 16 small slits into the flesh of the lamb. Insert half a clove of garlic into each slit. Rub the lamb with the olive oil, then sprinkle with the rosemary, thyme, and salt and plenty of freshly ground pepper. Place the lamb, fat side up, on a rack in a roasting pan. Set the pan in the oven and roast for 1¼ to 1½ hours. Baste several times during cooking with the accumulated juices. After 1 hour, start testing for doneness with a meat thermometer: 130°F for medium-rare, 140°F for medium. As soon as the lamb is done, remove it from the roasting pan and set aside for carving.

Pour off most of the fat from the roasting pan, reserving about 3 tablespoons to make the sauce. Place the roasting pan on top of the stove over high heat. When the pan is hot, add the stock and wine, scraping the browned bits from the bottom of the pan to release the flavors. Reduce the sauce by one-half. Turn off the heat and add the butter, 1 tablespoon at a time, swirling until melted and combined. Spoon the sauce over the carved meat. SERVES 8 TO 10

grilled butterflied leg of lamb

PROTEIN, HEALTHY FATS, VEGETABLES

DETOX, LEVEL 1, LEVEL 2

In a small dish, mix the chopped garlic, rosemary, salt, pepper, and olive oil. Place the lamb in a roasting pan and rub all over on both sides with the garlic–olive oil mixture. Squeeze the juice from the lemons all over the lamb. Let marinate at least 1 hour (best to marinate overnight) in a nonreactive container, covered and refrigerated. Make sure to take the meat out and let sit at room temperature for about 15 minutes before grilling.

Heat a grill to high heat.

Place the lamb on the hot grill and sear on each side for 5 to 7 minutes. This seals all the juices inside. Turn the heat down to medium and cook, turning often, for another 35 to 40 minutes. (If the grill has a cover, close it during cooking to roast the insides.) Check for doneness with a meat thermometer: 130°F for medium rare, 140°F for medium. Remove from the grill and let stand for 10 minutes before carving. Carve into thin slices and serve immediately. SERVES 10 TO 12

6 garlic cloves, chopped

3 tablespoons chopped fresh rosemary

2 tablespoons sea salt

Freshly ground black pepper

3 tablespoons olive oil

One 7- to 8-pound leg of spring lamb, boned and butterflied

Juice of 1½ lemons

lamb loin with tarragon salsa

PROTEIN, HEALTHY FATS, VEGETABLES

DETOX, LEVEL 1, LEVEL 2

2 medium tomatoes, diced

7 tablespoons extra virgin olive oil, plus more for the pan

2 tablespoons white wine vinegar

1 tablespoon chopped fresh tarragon

1 teaspoon sea salt

1/2 teaspoon freshly ground black pepper

2 pounds loin of lamb

In a medium bowl, combine the tomatoes, 5 tablespoons olive oil, vinegar, tarragon, ½ teaspoon salt, and ¼ teaspoon pepper. Set aside.

Preheat the oven to 375°F.

Rub the remaining 2 tablespoons oil, ½ teaspoon salt, and ¼ teaspoon pepper on the lamb.

Heat an ovenproof skillet on high heat. Add a little more olive oil to cover bottom of the pan. Place the lamb in the hot skillet and brown on all sides, about 5 minutes. Place the skillet in the oven and roast until a meat thermometer reaches 130°F for medium rare, 20 to 25 minutes. Remove from the oven and let the roast rest for 10 minutes. Slice the lamb on the diagonal and serve with a mound of salsa. SERVES 4

medallions of lamb with tomato and basil

PROTEIN, HEALTHY FATS, VEGETABLES

DETOX, LEVEL 1, LEVEL 2

2 racks of lamb, boned and trimmed

Sea salt and freshly ground black pepper

4 tablespoons ground cumin

2 tablespoons (1/4 stick) unsalted butter

4 tablespoons olive oil

12 to 15 shallots, chopped

6 garlic cloves, chopped

6 ripe medium tomatoes, chopped

1 bunch basil, leaves julienned

Slice the fillet of lamb into ½-inch medallions. Rub both sides of the medallions generously with salt, pepper, and cumin. Set aside.

Heat a large sauté pan over medium heat. Add the butter, 2 tablespoons of the olive oil, and the shallots. Sauté the shallots until they are lightly browned, about 2 minutes. Add the garlic and cook for 1 minute longer. Add the tomatoes, salt, and pepper. Lower the heat and simmer for 5 minutes.

In another pan, sauté the lamb medallions in the remaining 2 tablespoons olive oil for approximately 2 minutes on each side. Just before serving, toss the basil into the tomato sauce and pour over the lamb medallions. Serve immediately. SERVES 6

grilled lamb chops with fresh herbs

PROTEIN, HEALTHY FATS, VEGETABLES

DETOX, LEVEL 1, LEVEL 2

In a large nonreactive shallow dish, mix the oil, garlic, wine, and herbs. Add the lamb chops, cover, and marinate in the refrigerator for 4 hours, turning the chops after 2 hours to marinate both sides.

Let the chops sit out at room temperature for 15 minutes before cooking. Heat a grill to medium high. Season the lamb chops with salt and pepper. Grill until medium rare, 2 to 3 minutes per side. Arrange on a platter in a fan pattern and garnish with rosemary and thyme sprigs.   SERVES 6

^{1}/2 cup olive oil

6 garlic cloves, chopped

^{1}/2 cup dry red wine (use beef stock for Detox)

1 bunch fresh rosemary, chopped

2 tablespoons chopped fresh thyme leaves

18 baby lamb chops, 1 inch thick

Sea salt and freshly ground black pepper

Fresh rosemary and thyme sprigs, for garnish

grilled marinated lamb chops with lemon

PROTEIN, HEALTHY FATS

DETOX, LEVEL 1, LEVEL 2

Place the lamb chops, oil, and lemon juice in a glass or other nonreactive bowl and marinate at room temperature for 30 minutes, turning from time to time. Remove the chops and set aside.

Preheat the grill to medium high. Grill the lamb chops 2 to 3 minutes per side, until golden brown and a little crusty on the edges. Season both sides with salt and pepper. Serve immediately with lemon wedges.   SERVES 4

12 rib lamb chops, ^{1}/2 inch thick

^{1}/4 cup olive oil plus extra for the pan

3 tablespoons fresh lemon juice

Sea salt and freshly ground black pepper

Lemon wedges, for garnish

grilled lamb chops with lavender lamb jus

PROTEIN, HEALTHY FATS, VEGETABLES

DETOX, LEVEL 1, LEVEL 2

2½ tablespoons
  unsalted butter

2 shallots, thinly sliced

1 cup dry red wine
  (use beef stock for
  Detox)

½ cup veal demi-glace
  (see Note, page 259)

¼ cup beef stock,
  preferably
  homemade
  (page 34)

4 sprigs fresh lavender,
  or 1 teaspoon dried,
  plus 4 sprigs for
  garnish

4 sprigs fresh rosemary,
  or 1 teaspoon dried

Sea salt and freshly
  ground black pepper

Extra virgin olive oil

4 loin lamb chops,
  2 inches thick

Place a small saucepan on medium heat. Add ½ tablespoon of the butter and the shallots; sauté until the shallots become golden and slightly caramelized, 15 to 20 minutes. Add the wine to deglaze the pan and reduce it by half. Add the veal demi-glace, stock, and 2 lavender sprigs and 2 rosemary sprigs or half the dried herbs. Bring to a boil, then reduce to a simmer until it reduces again by half. Whisk in the remaining 2 tablespoons butter. Remove the herb sprigs. Adjust the seasoning with salt and pepper as needed.

Heat the grill to high.

Drizzle olive oil on the lamb chops. Season liberally with salt and pepper. Remove the stems from 2 sprigs lavender and the remaining rosemary and sprinkle the leaves (or dried herbs) onto the chops. Grill for 4 minutes per side for medium rare.

Place 2 chops onto each plate and generously spoon sauce over the top. Garnish each plate with 2 crisscrossed sprigs of lavender and serve immediately.   SERVES 2

baby lamb chops with parmesan crusts and sweet tomato sauce

PROTEIN, HEALTHY FATS, VEGETABLES

DETOX, LEVEL 1, LEVEL 2

4 large eggs, lightly beaten

12 rib lamb chops, 1/2 inch thick

1 cup freshly grated Parmesan cheese

Sea salt and freshly ground black pepper

1 bunch fresh thyme, or 2 tablespoons dried

3 tablespoons olive oil

Sweet Tomato Sauce (page 183)

Place the eggs in a large mixing bowl. Add the lamb chops and coat with egg. Place the Parmesan in a shallow bowl. Dip each chop into the cheese, coating both sides. Sprinkle both sides of the chops with salt, pepper, and thyme. Place chops in the refrigerator for a couple of hours to allow the "breading" to set. (Omit this step if time does not permit.) Let the chops sit out at room temperature before cooking (about 15 minutes).

Heat a large skillet, then add the olive oil to cover bottom of pan.

Cook the chops until the crusts are golden, then turn over to fry the other side, 2 to 3 minutes per side.

To serve, spoon 2 or 3 tablespoons of tomato sauce in the center of each plate. Arrange 3 chops per person on top of sauce. Serve immediately. SERVES 4

lamb shanks with oregano and feta

PROTEIN, HEALTHY FATS, VEGETABLES, CARBOHYDRATES

DETOX, LEVEL 1, LEVEL 2

4 lamb shanks

Sea salt and freshly ground black pepper

$^1/_2$ cup olive oil

3 medium onions, thinly sliced

6 cups chicken stock or broth, preferably homemade (pages 30–32)

3 tablespoons chopped fresh oregano leaves, or 2 tablespoons dried

$^1/_4$ teaspoon cayenne

One 28-ounce can peeled tomatoes, chopped, with juice

2 cups prepared whole wheat couscous (for Level 1 and Level 2 only)

8 ounces crumbled feta cheese

Trim any excess fat from the shanks, then season with salt and pepper. Heat the oil in a stockpot over high heat. Add the shanks, turning frequently to brown all sides. Remove from the pot and reserve.

Lower the heat to medium and add the onions, stirring until golden brown, 12 to 15 minutes. Add the stock, oregano, cayenne, and tomatoes with juice. Scrape the browned bits off the bottom of the pan to release the flavor. Add the shanks back to the pan. (If the shanks are not completely covered by liquid, add enough water to cover.) Bring to a boil, then lower the heat and simmer for about 2½ hours. The shanks are done when the meat is practically falling off the bone.

To serve, place about ½ cup couscous in the bottom of each serving bowl. Add a shank to each bowl and top with some sauce. Sprinkle with feta cheese and serve immediately. SERVES 4

lamburgers

PROTEIN, HEALTHY FATS, VEGETABLES

DETOX, LEVEL 1, LEVEL 2

Heat a grill to medium high. Place the lamb, salt, onion, egg, cumin, allspice, cayenne, and cilantro into a food processor and process until well blended (or mix by hand). Shape the mixture into 4 to 6 patties. Cook on a hot grill or in a frying pan for 5 minutes per side, or until they are well browned and cooked to your liking.

Serve patties with the red onion slices and a spoonful of crème fraîche or sour cream. Put a lemon wedge on each plate and serve immediately. MAKES 4 TO 6 BURGERS

1½ pounds ground lamb

1 teaspoon sea salt

1 onion, finely chopped

1 large egg, beaten

2 teaspoons ground cumin

½ teaspoon ground allspice

½ teaspoon cayenne

4 tablespoons coarsely chopped fresh cilantro leaves

1 red onion, thinly sliced

Crème fraîche (page 149) or sour cream

2 lemons, cut into wedges

herb-roasted loin of pork with warm cranberry relish

PROTEIN, HEALTHY FATS, FRUIT
DETOX, LEVEL 1, LEVEL 2

One 4-pound loin of
pork, with ribs

Olive oil

Sea salt and freshly
ground black pepper

1 bunch fresh marjoram

1 bunch fresh thyme

1 bunch fresh sage

1/2 cup dry red wine
(use stock for Detox)

1 cup veal demi-glace
(see Note, page 259)

1/4 cup chicken stock
or broth, preferably
homemade (pages
30–32)

2 tablespoons (1/4 stick)
unsalted butter

Warm Cranberry Relish
(recipe follows; omit
for Detox)

Preheat the oven to 450°F.

Rub the pork with olive oil, then season liberally with salt and pepper. In a large sauté pan over high heat, add the oil to coat the pan and sear the pork on all sides, 2 to 3 minutes on each side, until golden brown all over.

Remove the pork from the sauté pan and place in a roasting pan, bone side down. Place the herbs all over the roast, tucking sprigs between bones and through the skin to hold in place. Place in the oven and roast for 15 minutes. Lower the heat to 350°F and continue roasting for approximately 45 minutes, or until the internal temperature on a meat thermometer reads 160°F. Remove the roast from the pan and set aside to rest.

Place the roasting pan on the stovetop over medium heat. Add the wine, scraping any browned bits off the bottom of the pan. Continue cooking until the wine is reduced by half. Add the veal demi-glace and chicken stock and cook until the mixture begins to boil, 7 to 10 minutes. When the sauce is thickened, turn off the heat and stir in the butter until combined.

Slice the pork roast into single-rib chops and spoon the pan drippings over the top. Serve immediately with cranberry relish.   SERVES 6

warm cranberry relish

HEALTHY FATS, FRUIT

LEVEL 2

    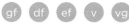

2 tablespoons olive oil

$^{1}/_{2}$ onion, finely diced

2 tablespoons finely minced fresh ginger

2 cups fresh whole cranberries

1 tablespoon sherry vinegar

$^{1}/_{3}$ cup All Natural SomerSweet

Sea salt and freshly ground black pepper

To a medium saucepan over medium heat, add the olive oil, onion, and ginger. Cook until the onion softens, 4 to 5 minutes. Add the cranberries, vinegar, All Natural SomerSweet, and ½ cup water. Cook until the berries pop and become soft, 10 to 15 minutes. Stir occasionally. Season to taste with salt and pepper. Serve immediately.   MAKES 1$^{1}/_{2}$ CUPS

chipotle-glazed pork with three salsas

PROTEIN, HEALTHY FATS, VEGETABLES, FRUIT

DETOX, LEVEL 1, LEVEL 2

1 whole pork tenderloin,
1½ to 2 pounds

2 tablespoons adobo
sauce, from canned
chipotle peppers

2 tablespoons olive oil,
plus more for the
pan

Sea salt and freshly
ground black pepper

1 cup Candied Tomato
Salsa (recipe follows)

Roasted Tomatillo Salsa
(recipe follows)

Mango Salsa (recipe
follows; for Level 2
only)

Place the pork in a medium glass or other nonreactive bowl. Mix the adobo sauce, oil, and salt and pepper; pour over the pork and cover. Marinate in the refrigerator for at least 1 hour, or overnight.

Let the pork sit out at room temperature for 15 minutes before cooking. Preheat the oven to 450°F.

Coat the bottom of an ovenproof sauté pan with olive oil. Place the pork in the pan and sear on all sides until nicely browned, about 4 minutes. Place in the oven and bake until cooked through, about 8 minutes. Remove from the oven and allow to rest before slicing.

Serve immediately with the salsas.   SERVES 2

candied tomato salsa

HEALTHY FATS, VEGETABLES

DETOX, LEVEL 1, LEVEL 2

6 Candied Tomatoes (page 174), coarsely chopped

1½ tablespoons extra virgin olive oil

1 tablespoon chopped fresh cilantro

1 red jalapeño or Fresno chile, finely chopped (see Note, page 39)

Sea salt and freshly ground black pepper

In a medium bowl, mix all the ingredients. Season with salt and pepper. Store in an airtight container in the refrigerator for up to 2 weeks.   MAKES 1 CUP

roasted tomatillo salsa

HEALTHY FATS, VEGETABLES

DETOX, LEVEL 1, LEVEL 2

6 tomatillos, husked, washed, and cut in half

2 tablespoons olive oil

Sea salt and freshly ground black pepper

Preheat the oven to 400°F.

Place the tomatillos on a rimmed baking sheet and drizzle with the olive oil, then sprinkle over salt and pepper. Roast until caramelized and soft, 35 to 45 minutes. Remove from the oven and while still warm, chop until they become the texture of chunky salsa. Serve warm or at room temperature. Store in an airtight container in the refrigerator for up to 2 weeks.   MAKES ABOUT ³/4 CUP

mango salsa

HEALTHY FATS, VEGETABLES, FRUIT

LEVEL 2

1 ripe mango, peeled, seeded, and diced

¹/2 red onion, finely diced

1 red jalapeño, seeds removed (see Note, page 39)

Juice from ¹/4 lime

1 tablespoon chopped fresh cilantro

1 tablespoon chopped fresh mint

1 tablespoon extra virgin olive oil

Sea salt and freshly ground black pepper

In a medium bowl, mix all the ingredients. Season with salt and pepper. Store in an airtight container in the refrigerator for 1 to 2 days.   MAKES 1 CUP

braised pork chops with purple cabbage

PROTEIN, HEALTHY FATS, VEGETABLES

DETOX, LEVEL 1, LEVEL 2

8 bone-in pork chops,
  ¹/₂ inch thick

Sea salt and freshly
  ground black pepper

4 tablespoons olive oil

4 cups shredded purple
  cabbage

¹/₂ cup chicken stock
  or broth, preferably
  homemade
  (pages 30–32)

1 cup port wine (use
  stock for Detox)

2 tablespoons balsamic
  vinegar

2 tablespoons (¹/₄ stick)
  unsalted butter

Season the pork chops with salt and pepper on both sides.

Place a large skillet over medium-high heat. Add 2 tablespoons of the olive oil and the cabbage. Stir-fry until tender, about 5 minutes. Remove from the pan and set aside in a warm oven.

Place the skillet back over medium-high heat. Add the remaining 2 tablespoons olive oil. Add the pork chops and cook for 5 to 6 minutes per side. Remove the chops from the pan and set aside with the cabbage. Add the stock, wine, and balsamic vinegar to the hot pan. Scrape all the browned bits from the bottom of the pan. Continue stirring until the sauce reduces by half. Turn off the heat and add the butter, 1 tablespoon at a time, until well combined.

Divide the cabbage among four plates. Top each with 2 pork chops. SERVES 4

pork tenderloin with sage

PROTEIN, HEALTHY FATS, VEGETABLES

DETOX, LEVEL 1, LEVEL 2

Place the pork tenderloins in a glass or other nonreactive container with the salt and pepper, olive oil, lemon juice, and chopped sage. Cover and refrigerate for at least 2 hours, turning after 1 hour.

Let the pork sit out at room temperature for 15 minutes before cooking. Preheat the oven to 350°F.

Place a large skillet (ovenproof, if possible) over medium-high heat. Remove the tenderloins from the marinade and sear in the hot pan, turning frequently until browned all over. If the skillet is ovenproof, place it in the oven and roast the tenderloins for 10 minutes. (If not, transfer the pork to a roasting pan, but use the skillet to make the sauce.)

When cooked, remove the pork from the skillet and set aside. Place the skillet over high heat. When hot, add the marsala. Cook until the steam evaporates. Add the stock and the 4 finely chopped sage leaves, scraping the bits off the bottom of the pan. Cook over high heat until the sauce reduces by half or more. Turn off the heat and stir in the butter. Season with salt and pepper.

Cut the tenderloins into ½-inch-thick strips on an angle. Arrange in a semicircle on a plate and serve with sauce. SERVES 4

2 whole pork tenderloins

Sea salt and freshly ground black pepper

1 cup olive oil

Juice of 1 lemon

2 teaspoons finely chopped fresh sage, or 1 teaspoon dried, plus 4 fresh sage leaves, finely chopped

1 cup marsala or white wine (use stock for Detox)

1 cup chicken stock or both, preferably homemade (pages 30–32)

2 tablespoons (¼ stick) unsalted butter

peppered pork chops with fried sage leaves

1 tablespoon black
  peppercorns

4 center-cut pork chops
  on the bone, about
  1 inch thick

Olive oil

Sea salt

1 bunch fresh sage
  leaves

PROTEIN, HEALTHY FATS

DETOX, LEVEL 1, LEVEL 2

Crack the peppercorns on a cutting board with a heavy pan.

Coat the pork chops with a drizzle of olive oil, then season them with the cracked peppercorns and sea salt. Place a large skillet on medium-high heat. Add about 2 tablespoons olive oil and the pork chops. Cook for 3 minutes on each side. Remove from the pan and set aside.

Add another 3 tablespoons olive oil to the pan and put over medium heat. After about 30 seconds, toss in the fresh sage leaves and sauté for 30 seconds. Remove with a slotted spoon and scatter over the pork chops. Season the fried sage leaves with a sprinkle of sea salt. SERVES 4

pork chops with creamy shallot sauce

PROTEIN, HEALTHY FATS, VEGETABLES

DETOX, LEVEL 1, LEVEL 2

4 boneless center-cut pork chops, 1 inch thick

Sea salt and freshly ground black pepper

4 tablespoons ($\frac{1}{2}$ stick) unsalted butter

1 medium onion, finely chopped

5 shallots, finely chopped

2 garlic cloves, chopped

1 cup dry red wine (use chicken stock for Detox)

$\frac{1}{2}$ cup heavy cream

Preheat the oven to 200°F.

Season the pork chops with salt and pepper. Heat a skillet on medium-high heat. Melt 2 tablespoons of the butter in the pan. Cook the chops for about 5 minutes, until the outside is golden brown. Turn them over and continue cooking for another 5 minutes. Remove the chops from the pan, and reserve in a warm oven.

Add the onion to the skillet (and more butter if the pan looks too dry) and cook until browned, about 7 minutes. Add the shallots and garlic, and cook for an additional minute. Pour the wine into the pan and bring to a boil. Turn the heat down to a simmer, and cook until the wine has reduced by half, 3 to 4 minutes. Add the remaining 2 tablespoons butter, stirring to melt. Whisk in the cream. Season with additional salt and pepper.

Return the pork chops to the pan, heat for 2 minutes in the sauce, and serve. SERVES 2

pork paillards with caper butter sauce

8 tablespoons (1 stick) unsalted butter, softened

4 boneless pork chops, (4 to 6 ounces each), pounded to $^1/_2$-inch thickness

Sea salt and freshly ground black pepper

2 tablespoons olive oil

$^1/_2$ cup finely chopped onion

$^1/_2$ cup chicken broth, preferably homemade (page 32)

2 tablespoons fresh lemon juice

2 tablespoons drained capers

Lemon slices, for garnish

Place a large sauté pan over medium-high heat. Add 4 tablespoons of the butter and swirl until melted. Season the pork chops with salt and pepper and sauté for 3 minutes. Turn and sauté an additional 3 minutes. Remove from the pan and transfer onto serving plates. Add the olive oil and onion to the pan. Sauté for 5 minutes, scraping any browned bits off the bottom of the pan. Add the broth and continue scraping the bits from the pan to release the flavor. Let reduce until thick and syrupy, about 5 minutes.

Reduce heat to low. Add remaining 4 tablespoons butter and stir until melted. Add the lemon juice and capers, and season with salt and pepper. Spoon the sauce over the pork chops. Garnish with lemon slices. SERVES 4

peppered pork tenderloin

PROTEIN, HEALTHY FATS
DETOX, LEVEL 1, LEVEL 2

Sprinkle the pepper on all sides of the tenderloin. Gently press the pepper into the pork. Slice the pork into ¼-inch-thick slices.

Place a large skillet over medium-high heat. Add 4 tablespoons of the butter and stir until melted. Add the pork and sauté for 2 minutes. Turn the pork over and sauté for an additional 2 minutes. Add the garlic to the pan and sauté for 30 seconds. Reduce the heat to low, add the brandy, and cook for 2 minutes. Add the remaining 4 tablespoons butter and stir until melted. Add the cream and heat until warm. Season with salt and pepper and serve. SERVES 4

NOTE If you are doing well on Level 1, the small amount of alcohol in this recipe is okay.

1 tablespoon coarsely ground black pepper

One 1½- to 2-pound pork tenderloin

8 tablespoons (1 stick) unsalted butter

3 garlic cloves, chopped

3 tablespoons brandy (omit for Detox; see Note)

¼ cup heavy cream

Sea salt and freshly ground black pepper

flattened pan-fried pork chops

PROTEIN, HEALTHY FATS, VEGETABLES
DETOX, LEVEL 1, LEVEL 2

Place the garlic, salt, peppercorns, and rosemary into a large shallow nonreactive container. Add the lemon juice and about ½ cup of olive oil. Add the chops, spooning the mixture over both sides of each chop. Leave in a cool place for about 1 hour.

Place a large skillet over medium-high heat. When the pan is hot, add 2 to 3 tablespoons olive oil. Add as many chops as will fit in the pan and fry for 5 to 6 minutes on each side. Repeat with the remaining chops.

Serve with lemon wedges. SERVES 8

6 garlic cloves

3 tablespoons sea salt

2 tablespoons black peppercorns, coarsely cracked

½ cup chopped fresh rosemary

Juice of 4 lemons

10 to 11 tablespoons olive oil

Eight 6-ounce boneless pork chops pounded to ½-inch thickness

8 lemon wedges

twelve-hour roast pork

1 whole pork shoulder pork with skin (7 to 9 pounds)

12 garlic cloves, finely chopped

One 1.6-ounce bottle fennel seeds

Sea salt and freshly ground black pepper

8 small dried red chiles, crumbled

Juice of 6 lemons

4 tablespoons olive oil

SAUCE

2 cups chicken broth, preferably homemade (page 32; optional)

Juice of 2 lemons (optional)

Preheat the oven to 450°F.

Score the entire skin of the shoulder by slicing deeply through the skin and into the meat. Continue scoring, making cuts ¼ inch apart from one another.

Place the garlic, fennel seeds, salt and pepper, and chiles in a food processor. Pulse until all the seasonings are coarsely ground. (If you do not have a food processor, chop by hand on a cutting board.) Rub this mixture all over the skin of the pork and into the cut areas to cover all surfaces of the meat.

Place the shoulder on a rack in a roasting pan and roast for 30 minutes, or until the skin begins to crackle and brown. Loosen the shoulder from the bottom of the pan and pour the juice of 3 lemons and 2 tablespoons of the olive oil over the pork.

Turn the oven temperature down to 250°F and slow-roast the pork for 12 to 18 hours. The pork becomes almost shredded, crispy on the outside and moist from the juices on the inside. It's ready when it is completely soft under the crisp skin. You can tell by pushing with your finger; the meat will give and might even fall off the bone. It will be cooked after 12 hours, but if you like it crispier, cook it for closer to 18 hours. Baste occasionally with the remaining lemon juice and olive oil.

If you would like to serve the pork with the pan drippings, remove the meat from the pan. Pour off most of the fat, leaving about 3 tablespoons. Place the roasting pan on the stove over medium heat. Scrape the browned bits as the pan heats up. When the pan gets hot, add the chicken broth and lemon juice. Deglaze the pan by scraping all the browned bits from the bottom of the pan. Reduce for about 5 minutes.

Serve shredded pork with a piece of the crisp skin. Spoon the sauce over the meat.   SERVES 15

NOTE The pork is also great served in lettuce cups or wrapped in warm whole wheat tortillas. Serve some salsa on the side.

traditional mexican carnitas

PROTEIN, HEALTHY FATS, VEGETABLES

DETOX, LEVEL 1, LEVEL 2

Cube the pork into 2½ × 2½-inch chunks. Place the pork in a large, shallow skillet and sprinkle with the salt. Barely cover with cold water and bring to a boil, uncovered. Lower the heat to medium and let the meat continue cooking briskly until all the liquid has evaporated—by this time it should be cooked through but not falling apart. Turn the heat down to medium low and continue cooking until all the fat has rendered out of the pork. The pork will begin to brown in its own juices. Keep turning until it is browned all over, about 70 minutes. The pork is done when it is a little crispy and shredding into pieces.

Remove the lettuce leaves from the head in whole pieces. Rinse and dry. Place a spoonful of meat in each lettuce leaf. Serve with salsa and sour cream. Fold up and eat like a taco. SERVES 6

1 boneless pork shoulder or butt (3 pounds), skin removed

2 teaspoons sea salt

1 head iceberg lettuce

Spicy Tomato Salsa (page 202) or a prepared version

One 16-ounce container sour cream

chile-braised pork with tomatillo salsa

PROTEIN, HEALTHY FATS, VEGETABLES

LEVEL 2

A 13-pound pork butt, cut into small chunks

Sea salt and freshly ground black pepper

2 tablespoons plus 2 teaspoons olive oil

1 red onion, medium diced

1 red bell pepper, seeded and medium diced

3 to 4 jalapeño chiles, sliced (see Note, page 39)

2 tablespoons tomato paste

1 cup chopped ripe tomato

2 cups chicken stock or broth, preferably homemade (pages 30–32)

$^1/_2$ jícama, peeled and finely julienned

$^1/_2$ red onion, thinly sliced

Juice from $^1/_2$ lime

1 tablespoon julienned fresh mint leaves

Tomatillo Salsa (recipe follows)

Tortilla Chips (recipe follows)

Season the pork with salt and pepper. In a braising pan (or stockpot) over medium-high heat, add the 2 tablespoons olive oil and the pork. Sear meat on both sides. Add the onion, red pepper, and chiles and allow to caramelize. Add the tomato paste, tomato, and stock. Bring to a boil and cover, reduce the heat to low, and cook until the pork falls apart, about 1 hour.

Remove the pan from the heat. Take out the pork, reserving the liquid in the pan, and allow the pork to cool. Pull the pork into small pieces and place in a bowl with ½ to ¾ cup of the liquid.

In a mixing bowl, combine the jícama, red onion, remaining 2 teaspoons olive oil, and the lime juice. Add salt and pepper to taste and set aside. Just before serving, add the mint and mix.

To serve, scoop a spoonful of salsa onto each tortilla chip, add a spoonful of the pork, and top with the jícama. Serve immediately.

SERVES 16

tomatillo salsa

HEALTHY FATS, VEGETABLES

LEVEL 2

1 yellow onion, finely diced

Olive oil

1 cup diced husked tomatillo

$^1/_2$ avocado, pitted and chopped

Sea salt and freshly ground black pepper

1 tablespoon chopped fresh mint

In a medium sauté pan over high heat, sauté the onion in a little olive oil until caramelized, about 5 minutes. Add the tomatillo and cook until soft, 5 or 6 minutes. Remove from the heat and put into a blender. Add the avocado and blend until smooth. Season with salt and pepper. Remove from the blender and fold in the mint. MAKES 1 CUP

tortilla chips

HEALTHY FATS, CARBOHYDRATES

LEVEL 2

Whole wheat tortillas
Coconut oil

Cut the tortillas into wedges or break into chip-size pieces. Pour the oil into a heavy pot until one-third full. Heat on high until the temperature reaches 375°F. Fry the tortillas, a few pieces at a time, until they bubble and float. Remove and drain on paper towels.

baby back pork ribs

PROTEIN, HEALTHY FATS, VEGETABLES

DETOX, LEVEL 1, LEVEL 2

6 racks baby pork ribs
(12 to 14 ribs each)

Olive oil

Sea salt and freshly
ground black pepper

1 bunch fresh thyme,
chopped, or
2 tablespoons dried

1 bunch fresh rosemary,
chopped, or
2 tablespoons dried

2 heads garlic, minced

Pinch of red pepper
flakes

1 large lemon

Preheat the oven to 375°F.

Fill a stockpot with water and bring to a rolling boil. Add the ribs and boil for 30 minutes.

Remove from the water and place ribs side by side in a large roasting pan. Liberally rub the ribs on both sides with olive oil and salt. Add pepper to both sides. Sprinkle the top side with thyme and rosemary. Add the minced garlic to cover ribs on top. Sprinkle more olive oil on top of the garlic to make the garlic crisp. Season with red pepper flakes to taste. Squeeze fresh lemon juice on top, and place the roasting pan in the hot oven. After about 15 minutes, carefully turn the ribs over to crisp the bottom side and cook for an additional 15 minutes. Then turn over once again and scrape up any of the garlic and herbs that have fallen off, and spoon on top of the ribs again. Cook for another 15 minutes. It should take a total of 45 minutes of cooking time. The ribs should look dark and crispy. Serve immediately, one rack per person. SERVES 6

jalapeño chili

PROTEIN, HEALTHY FATS, VEGETABLES

DETOX, LEVEL 1, LEVEL 2

1 pound hot Italian sausages,
cut into 1-inch lengths

1 pound sweet Italian
sausages, cut into
1-inch lengths

¼ cup olive oil

2 cups coarsely chopped
onions

6 garlic cloves, minced
(3 tablespoons)

2 pounds ground beef chuck

2 red bell peppers, cored,
seeded, and coarsely
chopped

6 jalapeño chiles, cored,
seeded, and cut into
⅛-inch dice (see Note,
page 39)

Three 35-ounce cans plum
tomatoes, drained (5 cups)

1 cup dry red wine (omit for
Detox)

1 cup chopped flat-leaf
parsley

2 tablespoons tomato paste

6 tablespoons chili powder

3 tablespoons ground cumin

2 tablespoons dried oregano

1 tablespoon dried basil

2 teaspoons salt

½ tablespoon fennel seeds

2 teaspoons freshly ground
black pepper

2 pounds ripe Roma (plum)
tomatoes, quartered

Grated Monterey Jack cheese,
for garnish

Sour cream, for garnish

Sliced scallions, white and
green parts

Place a large, heavy skillet over medium heat, and sauté the sausages until well browned. Transfer the sausages to paper towels to drain.

Heat a Dutch oven or heavy stockpot with the oil over medium heat. Add the onions and garlic, and cook until just wilted, 5 minutes. Raise the heat to medium high, and crumble in the ground chuck. Cook, stirring frequently to break up the pieces, until the meat is well browned.

Add the drained sausages, the red peppers, and the jalapeño to the mixture. Cook, stirring frequently, until the chiles are slightly wilted, 10 minutes.

Stir in the canned tomatoes, wine, parsley, tomato paste, and all the herbs and spices. Cook for about 10 minutes, stirring frequently. Then add the fresh tomatoes and cook another 10 minutes.

Serve the chili in bowls, with cheese, sour cream, and scallions on the side. SERVES 8 TO 10

desserts

for the serious sweet tooth

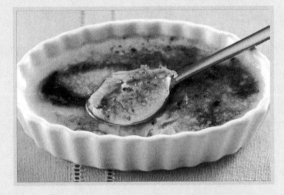

This girl has a sweet tooth . . . a serious sweet tooth! Figuring out how to eat sweets, while giving up sugar to control my weight, has been the crowning achievement of *Sexy Forever*. I'm certain it's the reason for the success of my program over the last fifteen years. I do not want to live in a world without chocolate, cream, caramel, custard, ice cream, and especially cake! And I'm sure you don't, either. So I have figured out how to have my cake and eat it, too.

I actually had a little tiff with my editor about how many dessert recipes to include here. She asked, "How can you have so many dessert recipes in a diet book?" *Sexy Forever* is not a diet! It's a lifestyle to teach you how to enjoy real, delicious food in moderate portions and still keep your figure.

Of all of the recipes from my Somersize books, the ones that need updating most are these dessert recipes, since All Natural SomerSweet did not exist when I first started writing that series of books. When I introduced SomerSweet, I started with a concentrated version, which was five times sweeter than sugar. The product has since been updated and now

All Natural SomerSweet is the same sweetness as sugar and easy to use spoon-for-spoon in coffee or tea, and also cup-for-cup in baking all of your favorite recipes. Since it's made with chicory fiber (a prebiotic fiber), it's actually good for your digestive system because it helps create healthy flora. You will find the correct measurements for All Natural Somer-Sweet in these updated pages.

You can make delicious Almond Chocolate Torte (page 327) with a high-quality chocolate (I always use at least 60 percent cocoa) and no added sugar. And Velvet Chocolate Pudding (page 319), Wild Berry Crostata (page 334), Lemon Curd Tart (page 332), and so many more!!! Whatever sweetener you choose—whether it's sugar, All Natural SomerSweet, or another of your liking—desserts are a thrill and I will continue my quest to show the world how to indulge without the bulge.

EGG SUBSTITUTIONS IN COOKING AND BAKING

For those allergic to eggs, here are some alternatives for baking I have been testing. Feel free to give them a try.

- 1 tablespoon milled flaxseed + 3 tablespoons water = 1 egg (Make sure that the mixture has gelled before using.)
- ¼ cup banana = 1 egg
- ¼ cup unsweetened applesauce = 1 egg
- 2 tablespoons water + 1 tablespoon oil + 2 teaspoons baking powder = 1 egg
- 2 tablespoons cornstarch = 1 egg
- 2 tablespoons arrowroot flour = 1 egg
- 2 tablespoons potato starch = 1 egg
- Egg white replacement: 1 tablespoon plain agar powder (available from health food stores) + 1 tablespoon water (Whip together, chill, then whip again.)

BAKING WITH ALL NATURAL SOMERSWEET

When using All Natural SomerSweet instead of sugar, I find it browns beautifully—unlike any other sugar substitute I have tried. In some cakes cooked at higher temperatures, the edges were getting too dark. This was easily remedied by lowering the baking temperature slightly, from 25° to 50°F. Feel free to adjust your own recipes accordingly.

decaf coffee granita

HEALTHY FATS

DETOX, LEVEL 1, LEVEL 2

8 cups strong decaffeinated coffee (for best results, use decaf espresso), cooled

1/2 cup All Natural SomerSweet or sugar, or to taste

Perfectly Whipped Cream (page 317; optional)

Combine the cooled coffee and the All Natural SomerSweet in a metal bowl. Place the bowl in the freezer. Every 30 minutes, open the freezer and use a metal whisk to stir the coffee, removing any frozen pieces from the side of the bowl. You will probably see the first frozen pieces after a couple of hours. Be sure to keep whisking your granita every 30 minutes until you are ready to serve it, or it will become one large ice block. After about 3 hours, the granita will be nicely frozen and ready to serve.

Spoon the granita into cups or glasses and top with whipped cream. SERVES 6

chocolate sorbet

INSULIN TRIGGERS

LEVEL 2

10 ounces dark chocolate (at least 60% cocoa)

1 cup brewed decaffeinated coffee

3 tablespoons All Natural SomerSweet or sugar

Chocolate Mint Leaves (page 326; optional)

Chop the chocolate into ½-inch pieces. Place in a food processor and process until finely chopped. Set aside.

Pour 1 cup water and the coffee into a small saucepan. Whisk in the All Natural SomerSweet and bring to a boil. Remove from the heat. With the food processor running, slowly pour the coffee mixture through the feed tube, melting the chocolate. Continue processing until the mixture is smooth. Pour the mixture into a bowl and allow to cool to room temperature, about 20 minutes. Cover and refrigerate for 2 hours.

Pour the mixture into an ice cream maker and freeze according to the manufacturer's directions. Scoop into pretty dishes and garnish, as desired, with chocolate leaves. SERVES 4

dark chocolate ice cream

PROTEIN, HEALTHY FATS, INSULIN TRIGGERS

LEVEL 1, LEVEL 2

Place the chocolate in a large mixing bowl and reserve.

Whisk egg yolks and vanilla in another mixing bowl until pale yellow, 3 to 4 minutes.

Warm the cream in a medium saucepan over medium heat to 110°F or until bubbles form along the edge, just before boiling. Slowly pour the hot cream into the egg yolks, stirring constantly. Return to the saucepan and stir over medium heat until the custard thickens or it coats the back of a spoon. Add the Somer-Sweet and stir until well combined. Pour the hot mixture over the chopped chocolate, stirring until smooth.

Allow the chocolate custard to cool to room temperature. Refrigerate it, loosely covered, a minimum of 3 hours. Transfer to an ice cream maker, and freeze according to the manufacturer's directions.　MAKES 3 PINTS

7 ounces unsweetened chocolate, chopped

5 large egg yolks

3 teaspoons vanilla extract

5 cups heavy cream

3/4 cup All Natural SomerSweet or sugar

vanilla bean ice cream

PROTEIN, HEALTHY FATS

DETOX, LEVEL 1, LEVEL 2

2¹/₂ cups heavy cream

2 vanilla beans, scraped, or 1 tablespoon vanilla extract

¹/₂ cup All Natural SomerSweet or sugar

8 large egg yolks

Pour ½ cup of the cream and ½ cup water into a large saucepan. To scrape the vanilla beans, use the tip of a sharp knife to split the vanilla beans lengthwise. Scrape out the little black seeds with the tip of the knife. Drop them into the cream. Add the All Natural SomerSweet, egg yolks, and vanilla bean pods. Over a double boiler, stir until combined and heated through. Do not boil. Add the remaining 2 cups of cream and stir until heated. Remove the vanilla bean pods. Pour into a bowl and place a piece of waxed paper over the top (right on top of the custard). Chill for 2 hours, then pour into an ice cream maker and freeze according to the manufacturer's instructions.

MAKES ABOUT 1 PINT

easy ice cream coffee treat

PROTEIN, HEALTHY FATS

DETOX, LEVEL 1, LEVEL 2

8 small scoops Vanilla Bean Ice Cream (above)

³/4 cup hot strong decaffeinated coffee

Place 2 scoops of the ice cream into four small bowls. Pour 3 tablespoons of the hot coffee over the top of each and serve immediately. SERVES 4

coffee ice cream

PROTEIN, HEALTHY FATS, CARBOHYDRATES

LEVEL 1, LEVEL 2

Heat 2 cups of the cream in a small saucepan over low until small bubbles appear around outer edge. (If you use an instant-read thermometer, the temperature of the cream should read about 120°F.) Remove from heat.

Place the yolks into the top of a double boiler over gently simmering water. Pour half of the hot cream over the egg yolks, stirring constantly. Cook until the mixture thickens slightly, about 4 minutes, or until a thermometer inserted into the mixture reads 160°F. Add the coffee, All Natural SomerSweet, and vanilla. Whisk until combined. Stir in the remaining 1 cup cream and the half-and-half. Refrigerate for 30 minutes. Freeze in an ice cream maker according to the manufacturer's directions.   MAKES 1 QUART

3 cups heavy cream

5 large egg yolks, lightly beaten

3 shots decaffeinated espresso or strong brewed coffee

1 cup All Natural SomerSweet or sugar

1 teaspoon vanilla extract

1 cup half-and-half

raspberry sorbet

FRUIT

DETOX, LEVEL 1, LEVEL 2

Place the raspberries, $^{1}/_{3}$ cup water, the All Natural SomerSweet, and lemon juice in a food processor or blender and blend until smooth. Place in an ice cream maker and freeze according to the manufacturer's directions.   MAKES ABOUT 2 CUPS

$2^{2}/_{3}$ cups fresh or frozen raspberries

$^{1}/_{2}$ cup All Natural SomerSweet or sugar

2 tablespoons fresh lemon juice

peach sorbet

FRUIT

DETOX, LEVEL 1, LEVEL 2

2^1/4 cups sliced peaches, fresh or frozen and thawed

^{3}/4 cup All Natural SomerSweet or sugar

2 tablespoons fresh lemon juice

Place the peaches, ^{1}/3 cup water, the All Natural SomerSweet, and lemon juice in a food processor or blender and blend until smooth. Taste and add more SomerSweet if needed. Place in an ice cream maker and freeze according to the manufacturer's directions.

MAKES ABOUT 3 CUPS

lemon crème fraîche ice cream

PROTEIN, HEALTHY FATS

DETOX, LEVEL 1, LEVEL 2

4 large egg yolks, beaten

3 cups crème fraîche (page 149) or sour cream, at room temperature

1 cup All Natural SomerSweet or sugar

Juice of 1 lemon

Pour the egg yolks into a stainless-steel bowl. Add 1 cup of crème fraîche, whisking constantly. Set aside. Place remaining 2 cups crème fraîche in a medium saucepan over low heat. Heat, stirring constantly, until warm; do not let crème fraîche boil. Slowly pour the warm crème fraîche into the egg mixture. Add the All Natural SomerSweet and lemon juice. Whisk well.

Place the bowl on top of a saucepan of simmering water. Whisk until mixture thickens and reads 170°F on an instant-read thermometer. Allow the mixture to cool to room temperature, about 30 minutes. Refrigerate for at least 2 hours, or overnight. Freeze in an ice cream maker according to the manufacturer's directions. MAKES 1 QUART

strawberry ice cream

PROTEIN, HEALTHY FATS, FRUIT

LEVEL 1, LEVEL 2

4 large egg yolks

$^1/_2$ cup half-and-half

2 cups heavy cream

One 16-ounce package
frozen strawberries,
or 2 cups fresh

$^3/_4$ cup All Natural
SomerSweet or
sugar

Place the egg yolks in a medium stainless-steel bowl and whisk for 2 to 3 minutes, until pale yellow. Set aside. Heat the half-and-half and cream in a small heavy-bottomed saucepan over medium heat until bubbles appear around the edge. Pour half of the hot cream mixture over the egg yolks, stirring constantly for 2 to 3 minutes. Add the remaining cream mixture and continue whisking for another minute.

Place the bowl over a saucepan of simmering water. Stir the egg-cream mixture for 3 minutes, until slightly thickened.

Place the strawberries into a food processor or blender. Pour the thickened egg-cream mixture over the fruit and allow the mixture to sit for 5 minutes. Add the All Natural SomerSweet. Pulse until the fruit is chopped but still chunky. If using fresh berries, chill the mixture for at least 2 hours, or overnight, then follow the ice cream maker instructions as directed. If using frozen berries, there is no need to chill the mixture. Freeze in an ice cream maker according to the manufacturer's directions. MAKES 1 QUART

bruce's café legois

HEALTHY FATS, CARBOHYDRATES, INSULIN TRIGGERS

LEVEL 2

6 ounces dark chocolate (at least 60% cocoa) broken up

$^3/_4$ cup heavy cream

1 pint Coffee Ice Cream (page 313)

$^1/_2$ cup hot decaf espresso or strong brewed decaf coffee

1 cup Perfectly Whipped Cream (page 317)

Chocolate-covered decaf espresso beans (optional)

Place the broken-up chocolate in a medium bowl. Pour the cream into a small saucepan and bring to a boil. Add the hot cream to the chocolate and stir until all the lumps are gone.

Place 2 scoops of coffee ice cream in each glass. Pour a little hot espresso over the top of each. Drizzle a little chocolate sauce over the top. Garnish with whipped cream and a couple of chocolate-covered espresso beans, if you like. Serve immediately. SERVES 4

dark chocolate fudge sauce

HEALTHY FATS, INSULIN TRIGGERS

LEVEL 1, LEVEL 2

6 ounces unsweetened chocolate, broken up

1$^1/_4$ cups heavy cream

2 tablespoons ($^1/_4$ stick) unsalted butter, softened

1$^1/_4$ cups All Natural SomerSweet or sugar

$^1/_2$ teaspoon vanilla extract

$^1/_2$ cup sour cream

Pinch of baking soda

Place the chocolate in a heavy-bottomed medium saucepan. Heat on low until the chocolate has melted. Add the cream and cook on medium heat, stirring constantly, until small bubbles appear around the edges or an instant-read thermometer inserted in the liquid reads between 90° and 100°F. Remove pan from heat.

Stir until the chocolate is dissolved and the mixture is smooth. The mixture will be thick. Add the butter and stir until smooth. Add the remaining ingredients and stir well. Use the fudge sauce while still warm, or refrigerate in an airtight container for up to 1 week.

MAKES 2 CUPS

raspberry coulis

HEALTHY FATS, FRUIT

DETOX, LEVEL 1, LEVEL 2

Place the raspberries, All Natural SomerSweet, and lemon juice in a food processor and pulse until pureed. Push the puree through a fine-mesh sieve to remove seeds. If you want the coulis thinner, adjust the consistency with 1 to 2 tablespoons water.

To serve warm, heat the strained puree in a saucepan, whisking in 1 to 2 tablespoons of unsalted butter, if using, for a glossy sheen.

MAKES 1 CUP

Two 6-ounce baskets fresh raspberries, or 12 ounces frozen, completely thawed

¼ cup All Natural SomerSweet or sugar

1 tablespoon fresh lemon juice

1 to 2 tablespoons unsalted butter (omit for Detox and Level 1)

perfectly whipped cream

HEALTHY FATS

DETOX, LEVEL 1, LEVEL 2

With an electric mixer, whip the cream until it starts to thicken. Add the vanilla and the All Natural SomerSweet. Continue whipping until soft peaks form. MAKES 4 CUPS

2 cups heavy cream

1 teaspoon vanilla extract

¼ cup All Natural SomerSweet or confectioners' sugar, to taste

chocolate pots de crème

PROTEIN, HEALTHY FATS, INSULIN TRIGGERS

LEVEL 2

2 cups heavy cream

4 ounces dark chocolate (at least 60% cocoa)

6 large egg yolks

2 tablespoons All Natural SomerSweet or sugar

Pinch of salt

1½ teaspoons vanilla extract

1 cup Perfectly Whipped Cream (page 317)

Preheat the oven to 325°F. Place 1½ cups of the cream in a small heavy saucepan over low heat. Place the remaining ½ cup cream and the chocolate in the top of a large double boiler over hot water on medium heat.

In a mixing bowl, lightly stir the yolks just to mix—do not beat.

When the cream is scalded (a slight skin will form on the top), stir in the All Natural SomerSweet and salt and remove from the heat.

Stir the chocolate mixture with a small wire whisk until perfectly smooth. Turn off the heat and very gradually add the hot cream to the chocolate, stirring constantly to keep the mixture smooth. Then gradually stir the chocolate mixture into the yolks and stir in the vanilla. Return the mixture to the top of the double boiler over hot water on low heat and cook, stirring constantly with a rubber spatula, for 3 minutes.

Pour the mixture through a fine strainer into a pitcher. Then pour it into the pots de crème cup or individual ramekins, leaving a bit of headroom. Place the cups in a shallow baking pan. Pour in hot water to about half the depth of the cups. Place the lids on top of the cups, or if using ramekins, place a cookie sheet over the top of the pan.

Bake for 22 minutes. The custard will look a little soft, but it will become firmer as it chills. It is best if it is still slightly creamy in the center when it is served. Remove the cups from the water and place on a rack to cool. Then refrigerate for a few hours. Serve with a spoonful of whipped cream. SERVES 6 TO 8

velvet chocolate pudding

PROTEIN, HEALTHY FATS, CARBOHYDRATES, INSULIN TRIGGERS

LEVEL 2

Place the oven rack in the middle position and preheat the oven to 275°F.

With the tip of a paring knife, scrape the seeds from the vanilla bean into a saucepan, then add the pod, the milk, cream, and All Natural SomerSweet and bring just to a boil, stirring until the SomerSweet is dissolved.

Add the chocolate and cook over moderately high heat, stirring gently with a whisk, until the chocolate is melted and the mixture just boils. Remove from the heat.

Pour the mixture into a metal bowl. Set the bowl into a larger bowl of ice and cold water and cool to room temperature, stirring occasionally, about 5 minutes.

Whisk in the yolks, then pour the entire mixture through a fine-mesh sieve. Discard the vanilla pod and any other solids.

Divide the mixture among six 4-ounce ramekins. Place the ramekins in a roasting pan. At the oven door, pour water into the roasting pan so that it comes halfway up the sides of the ramekins. Bake until the puddings are just set around the edge but the centers wobble when the ramekins are gently shaken, about 1 hour.

Cool the puddings in the water bath for 1 hour, then remove from the water and chill, uncovered, until cold, at least 1 hour.   SERVES 6

1/2 vanilla bean, halved lengthwise

1 1/2 cups whole milk

1/2 cup heavy cream

1/3 cup All Natural SomerSweet or sugar

5 ounces dark chocolate (at least 60% cocoa), roughly chopped

5 large egg yolks

vanilla custard

8 large egg yolks,
   beaten

2 tablespoons
   cornstarch

1 1/2 cups heavy cream

1/2 cup All Natural
   SomerSweet or
   sugar

1/2 teaspoon vanilla
   extract

Combine the egg yolks and cornstarch in a medium stainless-steel bowl. Pour the cream into a heavy-bottomed saucepan. Heat the cream on low heat until small bubbles appear around the outside edge or until an instant-read thermometer inserted reads 120°F. Slowly pour the cream over the eggs, stirring constantly.

Place the bowl of eggs and cream over a saucepan of simmering water. Cook for 4 to 5 minutes, stirring constantly until the mixture thickens, or until an instant-read thermometer inserted in the custard reads 160°F.

Add the All Natural SomerSweet and vanilla. Stir until the Somer-Sweet dissolves. Cover the surface with a piece of waxed paper. Allow the custard to cool to room temperature, about 1 hour. Refrigerate for at least 2 hours or until set. MAKES ABOUT 2 CUPS

crème brûlée

PROTEIN, HEALTHY FATS

DETOX, LEVEL 1, LEVEL 2

6 large egg yolks

$1/2$ cup All Natural SomerSweet or sugar

$2^1/4$ cups heavy cream

1 vanilla bean, split lengthwise and scraped

Preheat the oven to 350°F. Lightly butter eight 3-ounce ramekins or heatproof custard cups.

Lightly whisk the egg yolks with ¼ cup All Natural SomerSweet in a mixing bowl until frothy.

Heat the cream in a small saucepan until just scalded. Whisk the hot cream into the egg mixture. Add the scrapings from the inside of the vanilla bean.

Pour the custard into the ramekins. Place the ramekins in a roasting pan. At the oven door, add hot water to the bottom of the pan until the water comes half-way up the sides of the ramekins. (This is a water bath, which helps keep the custard from curdling, cracking, or breaking.) Bake until the custard starts to set up, about 20 minutes. Remove the ramekins from the water bath. Cover with waxed paper and refrigerate until firm, about 2 hours.

When ready to serve, sprinkle the remaining ¼ cup SomerSweet evenly over the tops of the custards. To caramelize the tops, use a kitchen propane torch or place the ramekins under a hot broiler, 3 inches from the heat, until the SomerSweet browns. SERVES 8

RASPBERRY CRÈME BRÛLÉE Using a 6-ounce basket of fresh raspberries, place as many raspberries as will fit side by side in the bottom of each ramekin. Proceed with Crème Brûlée instructions above.

lemon-scented ricotta

HEALTHY FATS, CARBOHYDRATES

LEVEL 1, LEVEL 2

1 cup heavy cream

2 cups whole-milk ricotta cheese

1/3 cup All Natural SomerSweet or sugar

2 tablespoons finely grated lemon zest

1 tablespoon fresh lemon juice

Place the cream in a mixing bowl and beat with an electric mixer until soft peaks form.

In another bowl, combine the ricotta, All Natural SomerSweet, half the lemon zest, and the lemon juice, and beat until fluffy, about 5 minutes.

Fold the whipped cream into the ricotta mixture until well incorporated. Spoon into custard cups and refrigerate overnight. Garnish with the remaining lemon zest before serving. SERVES 6 TO 8

lemon zabaglione

PROTEIN

DETOX, LEVEL 1, LEVEL 2

4 large eggs

4 large egg yolks

3/4 cup All Natural SomerSweet or sugar

1/2 cup fresh lemon juice (about 4 lemons)

Heat 1 inch of water to a simmer in a 3-quart saucepan (or the bottom of a double boiler). Place the eggs, egg yolks, and All Natural Somer-Sweet in a medium stainless-steel bowl (or the top of the double boiler) and add the lemon juice. Place the bowl over the simmering water. Whisk vigorously to combine, until the eggs are light and foamy and have thickened, 8 to 9 minutes.

Serve immediately, in small dishes or glasses. SERVES 6

COLD CREAMY LEMON ZABAGLIONE Instead of serving warm, let it cool to room temperature and add 3/4 cup heavy cream that has been whipped to soft peaks. Chill and serve.

chocolate fondue

HEALTHY FATS, FRUIT, INSULIN TRIGGERS

LEVEL 1, LEVEL 2

Place the warm fudge sauce into a fondue pot. Serve with the fresh berries. SERVES 6 TO 8

1 recipe Dark Chocolate Fudge Sauce (page 316)

1 pint fresh strawberries

1 pint fresh blackberries

1 pint fresh raspberries

warm chocolate soufflé cakes

PROTEIN, HEALTHY FATS, CARBOHYDRATES, INSULIN TRIGGERS

LEVEL 2

In a medium saucepan, melt the chocolate and butter over low heat. Set aside to cool.

In a medium bowl, combine the All Natural SomerSweet and cornstarch. In a separate bowl, whisk the eggs and yolks.

Add the eggs to the cooled chocolate mixture and stir until smooth. Add the SomerSweet mixture a little at a time, stirring to combine. Refrigerate overnight.

Preheat the oven to 400°F. Grease four 6-ounce mini cake molds or porcelain ramekins with butter.

Scoop the mixture into the molds, filling them two-thirds full. Bake for 20 minutes on the top rack in the oven, until set. They should spring lightly to the touch. Serve warm with whipped cream. SERVES 4

4 ounces dark chocolate (at least 60% cocoa)

6 tablespoons (^{3}/4 stick) unsalted butter, plus more for greasing

1 cup All Natural SomerSweet or sugar

1^3/4 tablespoons cornstarch

2 large eggs

2 large egg yolks

2 cups Perfectly Whipped Cream (page 317)

molten chocolate cakes

9 ounces dark chocolate (at least 60% cocoa)

11 tablespoons unsalted butter

3 large eggs

3 large egg yolks

1/2 cup All Natural SomerSweet or sugar

1/4 cup whole wheat pastry flour

2 cups Perfectly Whipped Cream (page 317)

Fresh raspberries, for garnish

Preheat the oven to 325°F. Butter 6 small glass custard cups, 3 to 4 ounces each.

In a double boiler, heat 6 ounces of the chocolate and the butter over 3 inches of simmering water until melted.

With the whisk attachment on the mixer, mix the eggs, yolks, and All Natural SomerSweet until pale and thick, about 10 minutes. Add the flour and melted chocolate and mix for 5 more minutes.

Pour the batter into the custard cups until almost half full. Chop the remaining chocolate and place in the center of the batter in each cup, then pour more batter on top, dividing the batter equally among the six cups.

Place the cups in the oven and bake for 12 to 15 minutes, until the sides seem stiff but the center jiggles when you touch it.

Cool for a few minutes. Slide a knife around the sides of the cups to make sure the cakes will slide out when flipped over. Invert each onto a plate and remove the cup. Prick the center with a fork and allow the chocolate to ooze out like lava. Serve with whipped cream and fresh raspberries.   SERVES 6

decadent chocolate cake

PROTEIN, HEALTHY FATS, CARBOHYDRATES, INSULIN TRIGGERS
LEVEL 2

Preheat the oven to 350°F. Butter and flour a 9-inch round cake pan.

For the cake: Melt the chocolate and butter in a double boiler (or in a bowl or smaller saucepan placed over a saucepan of boiling water). Set aside to cool.

Beat the egg yolks until light and fluffy, about 7 minutes. Slowly add the All Natural SomerSweet and continue beating until mixture is pale yellow. Fold in the melted chocolate. Sift the flour over the chocolate mixture until it just disappears.

In a separate bowl, whisk the egg whites until soft peaks form. Fold the egg whites into the chocolate mixture in two parts. Pour the batter into the prepared pan and tap on the counter to remove air bubbles. Bake for 20 to 25 minutes, until a toothpick comes out clean.

For the ganache: Place the chopped chocolate in a mixing bowl. Place the cream in a saucepan and bring to a boil. Add the hot cream to the chocolate and stir until all lumps are gone. Let the ganache stand until it reaches room temperature, then pour it over the cooled cake and spread with a spatula.   SERVES 6 TO 8

CAKE

7 1/2 ounces dark chocolate (at least 60% cocoa), chopped

11 tablespoons unsalted butter

4 large eggs, separated

1/3 cup All Natural SomerSweet or sugar

1/3 cup whole wheat pastry flour

CHOCOLATE GANACHE

6 ounces dark chocolate (at least 60% cocoa), chopped

3/4 cup heavy cream

chocolate mint leaves

INSULIN TRIGGERS

LEVEL 1, LEVEL 2

6 ounces dark
chocolate (at least
60% cocoa)

30 fresh mint leaves
with leaf stems,
cleaned and dry

Melt the chocolate in a double boiler or a heatproof bowl set over a saucepan of simmering hot water, stirring constantly, making sure the chocolate does not get too warm. Remove the bowl from the heat and continue to stir until the chocolate is melted and smooth as silk.

Place a piece of parchment or waxed paper on a cookie sheet. Place a rolling pin, covered with parchment, on the paper.

Take a mint leaf by its stem and dip it into the chocolate. Place the leaf on the rolling pin to dry. Be sure you coat both sides of the mint leaf, then brush the stem with chocolate. Putting it on a rolling pin causes the leaf to dry with a natural curl to it. Complete these steps with the remainder of the chocolate.

Place the leaves into the freezer to set. When dry and frozen, put them in an airtight container and use as needed. They keep well for 1 week.   MAKES ABOUT 30 LEAVES

almond chocolate torte

PROTEIN, HEALTHY FATS, CARBOHYDRATES, INSULIN TRIGGERS

LEVEL 2

Preheat the oven to 350°F. Butter an 8-inch round springform pan. Line the bottom with buttered waxed paper.

Grind the almonds in a food processor. Add the chocolate and pulse until the mixture is uniformly ground.

Cream the butter and All Natural SomerSweet together with an electric mixer until light and pale. Add the egg yolks one by one, mixing well between each addition. Then add the chocolate and nut mixture, blending until just combined.

In a separate bowl, beat the egg whites until they form soft peaks. Using a spatula, fold one-fourth of the egg whites into the chocolate mixture with large circular motions. Now take this chocolate mixture and fold it into the remaining egg whites.

Pour the batter into the prepared pan. Bake for 35 to 40 minutes. Cool on a rack for 30 minutes. Release the springform, slice, and serve with whipped cream.   SERVES 8 TO 10

1¹/₂ cups whole blanched almonds

8 ounces dark chocolate (at least 60% cocoa), broken into pieces

1 cup (2 sticks) unsalted butter, softened

¹/₂ cup All Natural SomerSweet or sugar

6 large eggs, separated

Perfectly Whipped Cream (page 317)

raspberry meringue cake

9 egg whites (about 1 cup), at room temperature

1½ cups All Natural SomerSweet or sugar

Pinch of sea salt

¼ cup Raspberry Coulis (page 317)

Perfectly Whipped Cream (page 317)

Preheat the oven to 250°F. Line a nonstick 8- or 9-inch round spring-form pan with waxed paper or parchment paper.

Place the egg whites in a clean stainless-steel bowl of an electric mixer. Beat on medium speed until frothy. Add the All Natural Somer-Sweet, ½ teaspoon water, and the salt. Increase the speed to high and beat until the egg whites form stiff peaks, about 6 minutes. Do not let the egg whites get too dry.

Spoon the meringue into the prepared pan. Distribute evenly over the bottom of the pan, taking care not to deflate the batter. Bake in the center of the oven for 1 hour.

Remove the cake from the oven and allow it to cool for 5 minutes. Carefully run a thin-bladed knife or metal spatula around the edge of the cake to loosen it. Remove the outside edge of the pan. Run a spatula underneath the cake to loosen it from the waxed paper underneath. Transfer the cake onto a serving platter.

Fold the coulis into the whipped cream. Using a spatula, smooth the mixture over top and sides of cake. Serve immediately or refrigerate. SERVES 6 TO 8

chocolate cupcakes with whipped cream filling

PROTEIN, HEALTHY FATS, CARBOHYDRATES, INSULIN TRIGGERS

LEVEL 2

Preheat the oven to 350°F. Grease a 12-cup muffin tin and set aside. Take 2 tablespoons of the flour and coat the muffin tin. Tap out excess flour.

For the cupcakes: Mix the remaining flour, All Natural SomerSweet, cocoa powder, baking powder, baking soda, and salt in a medium bowl.

In a separate bowl, beat the egg whites until frothy. Add the mayonnaise, vanilla, cream, 1 cup water, and the coffee granules. Whisk until well blended.

Pour the wet mixture into the dry ingredients and stir thoroughly until the batter is smooth. Divide the batter among the muffin tins. Bake for 12 to 15 minutes, or until a toothpick inserted into the center comes out clean. Cool on a wire rack for 10 minutes. Remove cupcakes from the muffin tins and cool completely before filling, about 20 minutes.

When cupcakes are cool, use a melon baller to scoop a hole from the bottom of each one. Reserve the piece of cake to use as a plug. Using the melon baller, enlarge the hole in the center of the cupcake. Set cupcakes aside.

For the filling: With an electric mixer, whip the cream until it starts to thicken. Add the vanilla and SomerSweet. Continue whipping until soft peaks form. Using a small spoon or butter knife, fill the cupcake holes with the whipped cream. Use the reserved cupcake bottoms to plug the holes. Place right side up on a piece of waxed paper.

For the frosting: Carefully reheat the sauce in a microwave on high for 30 seconds. Stir well. Repeat heating and stirring until mixture is smooth. Do not overheat or sauce will separate. Spoon sauce carefully over tops of cupcakes. MAKES 12

CUPCAKES

$1^{1}/3$ cups whole wheat flour

2 cups All Natural SomerSweet or sugar

$^{2}/3$ cup unsweetened cocoa powder

1 teaspoon baking powder

1 teaspoon baking soda

$1^{1}/2$ teaspoons sea salt

3 large egg whites

$^{2}/3$ cup mayonnaise

2 teaspoons vanilla extract

$^{1}/3$ cup heavy cream

2 tablespoons instant decaffeinated coffee granules

FILLING

$^{2}/3$ cup heavy cream

$^{1}/2$ teaspoon vanilla extract

2 tablespoons All Natural SomerSweet or sugar

FROSTING

Dark Chocolate Fudge Sauce (page 316)

mini coconut baked alaska

PROTEIN, HEALTHY FATS, INSULIN TRIGGERS

LEVEL 2

COCONUT ICE CREAM

2 1/2 cups heavy cream

8 large egg yolks

3/4 cup All Natural SomerSweet or sugar

1 cup coconut milk

CRUST

10 ounces dark chocolate (at least 60% cocoa), chopped

3 ounces unsweetened chocolate, chopped

12 tablespoons (1 1/2 sticks) unsalted butter

5 large eggs, at room temperature

1/2 cup All Natural SomerSweet or sugar

MERINGUE

4 large egg whites

2/3 cup All Natural SomerSweet or sugar

1/2 teaspoon vanilla extract

For the ice cream: Pour the cream and ½ cup water into a heavy saucepan. Heat until hot, but not boiling; remove from the heat. Place the yolks in a medium bowl. Whisk for 2 minutes. Pour the cream over the eggs, whisking constantly. Pour the mixture back into the saucepan and place over low heat. Stir until the mixture thickens and coats the back of a spoon. Pour the mixture through a sieve into a clean bowl. Add the All Natural SomerSweet and coconut milk. Stir well. Cover and cool to room temperature. Refrigerate for at least 2 hours. Pour into an ice cream machine and freeze according to the manufacturer's directions.

For the crust: Preheat the oven to 350°F. Butter six 6-ounce ramekins and set aside.

Melt the chocolates and butter together in a double boiler over gently simmering water. Stir until the chocolate is smooth. Remove from the heat and allow the mixture to cool slightly. Meanwhile, beat the eggs until pale and tripled in volume, 8 to 10 minutes. Add the All Natural SomerSweet and beat for another minute. Mix one-third of the egg mixture into the chocolate mixture; carefully fold the rest of the egg mixture into the chocolate. Pour into prepared ramekins. Bake for 17 minutes. Cool completely, then refrigerate for at least 1 hour.

Place ¼ cup ice cream inside each ramekin; flatten and smooth the top. Cover with waxed paper and freeze.

For the meringue: Preheat the oven to 400°F. Beat the egg whites in a mixer until soft peaks form. Add the All Natural SomerSweet and vanilla, and beat until stiff peaks form. Dollop on top of the frozen ice cream. Place in the hot oven for 5 minutes, or until the meringue is golden brown. Cool for 5 minutes. Serve within 5 minutes. SERVES 6

berry pie

HEALTHY FATS, CARBOHYDRATES, FRUIT, INSULIN TRIGGERS
LEVEL 2

Preheat the oven to 400°F.

Mix the cornstarch with the orange juice until smooth. Add the All Natural SomerSweet and blend until well combined. Gently toss the berries with this mixture and let sit for about 15 minutes.

Grease a 9-inch pie pan and line it with one piece of dough. Pierce the dough with a fork in several places. Bake for 7 to 10 minutes, or until the crust is lightly browned. Remove the pie pan and turn up the oven to 450°F.

Place the berries in the bottom crust. Cover with the second piece of dough, making slits to let out the steam (or make a lattice top, if you prefer). Bake for 10 minutes. Reduce the heat to 350°F and bake for 45 minutes more, until juices are thickened and bubbly. Cool for a few hours before cutting and serving. SERVES 6 TO 8

2 tablespoons cornstarch

1/4 cup orange juice

1/3 to 1/2 cup All Natural SomerSweet or sugar, depending on sweetness of berries

6 cups fresh or frozen berries (raspberries, blackberries, blueberries)

Whole Wheat Tart Crust (page 335), unbaked

lemon curd tart

PROTEIN, HEALTHY FATS, CARBOHYDRATES, INSULIN TRIGGERS

LEVEL 2

3 tablespoons unsalted butter, softened

¼ cup agave or honey

2 large eggs, lightly beaten

¼ cup fresh lemon juice

Grated rind of 2 lemons

1 prebaked 9-inch Whole Wheat Tart Crust (page 335), cooled

Mint sprig or small edible flowers (pansies or nasturtium), for garnish

Blend the butter and the agave in a double boiler (or in a bowl or smaller saucepan placed over a saucepan of boiling water). When well combined, mix in the eggs, stirring constantly. Add the lemon juice and rind. Continue stirring until the custard thickens and coats the back of a wooden spoon.

Fill the crust with the lemon curd and garnish with a sprig of mint or flowers. Set aside until the curd is set. Tastes best when served at room temperature. SERVES 6 TO 8

fresh berry custard tart

PROTEIN, HEALTHY FATS, CARBOHYDRATES, FRUIT, INSULIN TRIGGERS

LEVEL 2

½ cup All Natural SomerSweet or sugar

¼ cup cornstarch

4 large egg yolks

2 cups whole milk

½ teaspoon vanilla extract

1 prebaked 9-inch Whole Wheat Tart Crust (page 335), cooled

2 cups mixed fresh berries, such as blackberries, raspberries, strawberries, or boysenberries

Combine ¼ cup of the All Natural SomerSweet and all of the cornstarch in a mixing bowl and blend with a fork until smooth. Add the egg yolks and ½ cup of the milk, forming a paste.

Put the remaining 1½ cups milk and remaining ¼ cup SomerSweet in a saucepan and bring to a boil. Add the hot milk mixture to the cold ingredients, whisking constantly. Pour back into the pan and stir over medium heat until smooth and thick. Remove from heat and add the vanilla. Chill for 2 hours.

Fill the cooled crust with the chilled custard. Arrange the berries in a pretty pattern on top, and serve. SERVES 6

strawberry-rhubarb cobbler

HEALTHY FATS, CARBOHYDRATES, FRUIT, INSULIN TRIGGERS

LEVEL 2

Preheat the oven to 350°F.

For the filling: In a large bowl, combine the strawberries, rhubarb, vanilla, All Natural SomerSweet, orange juice, and cornstarch. Mix well and set aside.

For the topping: In a stand mixer fitted with a paddle (or in a bowl), combine the flour, All Natural SomerSweet, baking powder, baking soda, and salt. Add the butter and mix until a coarse mixture (or cut the butter into the dry ingredients with a pastry cutter or two knives). Add the buttermilk and, using a fork, mix until a dough forms. Turn out onto a work surface and knead gently, but do not overwork.

Roll the dough out until it is ½ inch thick, adding flour as needed. Using a cookie cutter, cut out biscuits and place on a cookie sheet while setting up the dish.

Place the fruit filling into a 9 × 13-inch baking dish and top with the biscuits. Bake for 30 to 40 minutes, until the fruit is bubbling and the biscuits are golden brown. Serve hot, topped with whipped cream or vanilla ice cream. SERVES 8

FILLING

4 cups fresh strawberries, hulled and quartered

4 cups chopped rhubarb (in 1-inch pieces)

1 teaspoon vanilla extract

1 cup All Natural SomerSweet or sugar

2 tablespoons orange juice

2 tablespoons cornstarch

2 cups Perfectly Whipped Cream (page 317) or vanilla ice cream

TOPPING

1⅓ cups white whole wheat flour (see Note, page 335) or whole wheat pastry flour

2 tablespoons All Natural SomerSweet or sugar

1¼ teaspoons baking powder

1 teaspoon baking soda

¼ teaspoon sea salt

4 tablespoons (½ stick) cold unsalted butter, cut up

½ cup buttermilk

strawberry gratin

HEALTHY FATS, FRUIT

LEVEL 1, LEVEL 2

4 cups fresh
strawberries

2 cups sour cream

1 tablespoon All Natural
SomerSweet or
sugar

2 teaspoons vanilla
extract

3 tablespoons All
Natural SomerSweet
or brown sugar

Preheat the broiler.

Wash the strawberries and slice off the end with the hull and stem. Place the berries, cut side down, sitting upright in a tart pan. Nuzzle them together, side by side, as many as will fit in the pan.

In a bowl, mix the sour cream, 1 tablespoon of the All Natural SomerSweet, and vanilla. Pour over the berries. Sprinkle the remaining 3 tablespoons SomerSweet (or brown sugar) over the strawberries and broil for 3 to 5 minutes, until the top gets brown and crusty. Serve warm.   SERVES 4

wild berry crostata

HEALTHY FATS, CARBOHYDRATES, FRUIT

LEVEL 1, LEVEL 2

4 cups mixed berries
(blackberries,
raspberries,
blueberries)

2 tablespoons All
Natural SomerSweet
or sugar

Zest of 1 lemon

Zest of 1 orange

Whole Wheat Tart
Crust (recipe
follows), unbaked

2 tablespoons (¼ stick)
unsalted butter

Preheat the oven to 425°F.

In a large bowl combine the berries, All Natural SomerSweet, and zests. Gently stir to combine.

Place the 2 pieces of rolled-out tart dough onto a baking sheet. Spoon half of the berries onto the center of each piece of dough. Bring the edges of the dough up around the sides of the fruit to create a crust that encloses the fruit but leaves the center open. Top each tart with a tablespoon of butter.

Bake for about 20 minutes, until the crust is golden and the center is bubbly. Cool for 15 minutes before cutting.   SERVES 8

whole wheat tart crust

HEALTHY FATS, CARBOHYDRATES

LEVEL 1, LEVEL 2

2¹/₂ cups white whole wheat flour (see Note) or whole wheat pastry flour

2 tablespoons All Natural SomerSweet or sugar

2 teaspoons sea salt

1 cup (2 sticks) unsalted butter, chilled

¹/₄ cup ice water

1 teaspoon vanilla extract

In a food processor, combine the flour, All Natural SomerSweet, and salt; pulse to blend. Add the butter and process to form crumbs. Sprinkle in the ice water and vanilla and process just until the dough forms a ball.

Remove the dough from the processor; divide in half and pat into two 1-inch-thick disks. Wrap each disk in parchment or waxed paper and refrigerate for at least 45 minutes. (The dough may also be frozen at this point and thawed for later use.)

For tarts that call for prebaked shells, preheat the oven to 425°F.

Remove the dough from the refrigerator. Place the dough pieces between two pieces of parchment paper, adding flour as necessary to avoid sticking. Roll each dough piece into a large round shape, about ¼ inch thick. Gently lay the dough over a rolling pin and very slowly flip each over into a well-greased tart pan. Press the dough into the pans gently and trim the edges to ¼ inch. Bake for about 10 minutes, or until golden brown. (For pies or crostatas, bake as specified in the recipe.)   MAKES TWO 9-INCH TART SHELLS

NOTE White whole wheat flour is a whole-grain flour made from the hard white kernel of wheat. Available at KingArthurFlour.com.

bittersweet chocolate citrus tart

LEVEL 2

CRUST

8 tablespoons (1 stick) unsalted butter, melted

1/2 cup All Natural SomerSweet or sugar

3/4 teaspoon vanilla extract

1 teaspoon sea salt

1 cup white whole wheat pastry flour (see Note, page 335)

FILLING

8 ounces dark chocolate (at least 60% cocoa), finely chopped

5 tablespoons unsalted butter, cut up

Zest of 1 tangerine

Zest of 1 ruby red grapefruit

1 large egg yolk

1/4 cup boiling water

For the crust: In a medium bowl, combine the butter, All Natural Somer-Sweet, vanilla, and salt. Slowly add the flour and stir until just blended. Press the dough into the bottom and sides of an 8-inch tart pan and chill for 30 minutes.

Preheat the oven to 350°F.

Remove the crust from the refrigerator and bake until deep golden brown, about 25 minutes. Cool in the pan on a rack.

For the filling: In a stainless-steel bowl, combine the chocolate, butter, and zests. Melt over a pan of simmering water.

In a separate bowl, whisk the egg yolk slowly with the boiling water. Cook over a pan of simmering water, stirring constantly, until the temperature reaches 160°F, about 3 minutes. Strain into the chocolate mixture and mix until smooth. Pour into the crust and refrigerate until ready to serve, at least 30 minutes. SERVES 6 TO 8

pear cobbler with chocolate crumble topping

HEALTHY FATS, CARBOHYDRATES, FRUIT, IINSULIN TRIGGERS
LEVEL 2

Preheat the oven to 375°F. Butter a 9 × 13-inch baking dish and set aside.

For the filling: Combine the pear slices, lemon juice, and almond extract in a large bowl. Add the All Natural SomerSweet and flour and toss to combine. Pour the filling into the prepared baking dish. Set aside.

For the topping: Mix the flour, oats, All Natural SomerSweet, and cinnamon in a medium bowl. Add the butter and rub in with your fingers until moist clumps form. Mix in the chopped chocolate.

Sprinkle the topping over the pear mixture. Bake until the topping is golden brown, 25 to 30 minutes. Cool at least 20 minutes before serving. Serve warm or at room temperature. SERVES 6

FILLING

3 pounds ripe pears, peeled, cored, and cut into 1/4-inch-thick slices, or 2 pounds frozen sliced pears, thawed and drained

1 tablespoon fresh lemon juice

1 1/2 teaspoons almond extract

1/2 cup All Natural SomerSweet or sugar

1 1/2 tablespoons white whole wheat flour (see Note, page 335) or whole wheat pastry flour

TOPPING

1/2 cup white whole wheat flour (see Note, page 335)

2/3 cup old-fashioned rolled oats

2 1/4 cups All Natural SomerSweet or sugar

1 teaspoon ground cinnamon

4 tablespoons (1/2 stick) unsalted butter, cut into 1/4-inch pieces

5 ounces dark chocolate (at least 60% cocoa), chopped into 1/4-inch pieces

cherry clafouti

1½ pounds fresh cherries (with pits), or 2 pounds frozen (see Note)

2 large eggs

1 large egg yolk

⅔ cup All Natural SomerSweet or sugar, plus more for dusting

5 tablespoons unsalted butter, melted

⅔ cup white whole wheat flour (see Note, page 335) or whole wheat pastry flour

1 cup heavy cream

Crème fraîche (page 149; optional)

Preheat the oven to 350°F. Butter a 9-inch round or square baking dish.

Wash, dry, and stem the cherries. Place them in the baking dish.

Combine the eggs and the yolk in a large bowl, add the All Natural SomerSweet, and whisk in the melted butter. Sift in the flour and mix well. Then mix in the cream and continue beating until the batter is smooth. Pour over the cherries.

Bake for 40 minutes, until golden brown. Remove from the oven and dust lightly with a little more SomerSweet. Serve lukewarm from the baking dish, with crème fraîche, if desired.   SERVES 8

NOTE Baking the cherries with their pits imparts a wonderful flavor. Be sure to warn your guests, though, so no one cracks a tooth.

mountain of lemon meringue pie

1 prebaked 9-inch Whole Wheat Tart Crust (page 335)

1 recipe Lemon Curd (page 332)

6 large egg whites

¼ teaspoon cream of tartar

1 cup All Natural SomerSweet or sugar

Fill the prepared pie crust with the lemon curd and chill to set.

Preheat the oven to 375°F.

Beat the egg whites with the cream of tartar until fluffy. Continue beating, gradually adding the All Natural SomerSweet, for 5 to 8 minutes, until stiff peaks form. Smooth the meringue over the lemon curd filling, covering it completely. Spoon the rest of the meringue onto the center of the pie. Using a spatula, draw the meringue upward so it resembles a mountain.

Bake for 7 to 10 minutes, or until the meringue is golden brown. Serve at room temperature. Do not chill.   SERVES 6 TO 8

decadent chocolate brownies

PROTEIN, HEALTHY FATS, INSULIN TRIGGERS

LEVEL 2

Preheat the oven to 350°F. Butter an 8-inch square baking pan and set pan aside.

Melt the chocolate and butter together in a double boiler over gently simmering water. Stir until chocolate is smooth. Remove from heat and allow the mixture to cool slightly.

Meanwhile, beat the eggs until pale and tripled in volume, 8 to 10 minutes. Add the All Natural SomerSweet and beat for another minute. Mix one-third of the egg mixture into the chocolate mixture. Carefully fold the rest of the egg mixture into the chocolate mixture.

Pour the batter into the prepared pan. Pour the fudge sauce on top of the brownie batter and swirl with a butter knife.

Bake for 35 minutes. The batter will not appear to be completely set. Cool completely before refrigerating, then refrigerate for at least 1 hour.

Cut into squares. Serve at room temperature.   MAKES 36 BROWNIES

14 ounces dark chocolate (at least 60% cocoa), chopped

12 tablespoons (1^1/2 sticks) unsalted butter

5 large eggs, at room temperature

^{3}/4 cup All Natural SomerSweet or sugar

^{1}/2 cup Dark Chocolate Fudge Sauce (page 316), warmed

chocolate soufflé with whipped cream and hot chocolate sauce

PROTEIN, HEALTHY FATS, INSULIN TRIGGERS

LEVEL 2

SOUFFLÉ

4 ounces dark chocolate (at least 60% cocoa)

3 large egg yolks

$^{1}/_{2}$ cup All Natural SomerSweet or sugar

5 large egg whites

HOT CHOCOLATE SAUCE

6 ounces dark chocolate (at least 60% cocoa), chopped

$^{3}/_{4}$ cup heavy cream

2 cups Perfectly Whipped Cream (page 317)

Preheat the oven to 400°F. Butter a 1-quart soufflé dish.

For the soufflé: Melt the chocolate in a double boiler (or in a bowl or smaller saucepan placed over a bigger saucepan of boiling water). In a bowl, beat the egg yolks until they are pale yellow, then add the All Natural SomerSweet. Continue to beat until well blended. Remove the chocolate from the heat and slowly add the egg mixture to the chocolate mixture. You don't want the eggs to cook.

In a separate bowl, beat the egg whites until they are stiff. Pour the chocolate mixture into the egg whites and fold in gently with a spatula, using wide circular motions so that you keep as much air in the mixture as possible. Gently pour the mixture into the buttered soufflé dish and bake for about 20 minutes.

For the chocolate sauce: Place the chopped chocolate in a bowl. Place the cream in a saucepan and bring to a boil. Add the hot cream to the chocolate and stir until all the lumps are gone.

When the soufflé is done, serve immediately with a spoonful of hot chocolate sauce and a dollop of whipped cream. SERVES 4 TO 6

tangerine soufflé with crème anglaise

PROTEIN, HEALTHY FATS, FRUIT

LEVEL 2

Preheat the oven to 400°F. Butter a 1-quart soufflé dish.

Pour the tangerine juice into a saucepan over medium-high heat. Let the juice reduce by three-fourths, until it becomes thick and syrupy. Remove from heat and set aside.

Beat the egg yolks and half of the All Natural SomerSweet until light and tripled in volume, 6 to 8 minutes. Add 2 tablespoons of the reduced tangerine syrup, the tangerine zest, and the cream. Continue to beat for another minute. Set aside.

In another bowl, beat the egg whites until frothy. Add the remaining All Natural SomerSweet and beat until stiff peaks form. Gently fold the egg whites into the yolk mixture until well incorporated. Transfer to the soufflé dish and bake for about 20 minutes. Serve immediately with tangerine crème anglaise. SERVES 4

1/2 cup tangerine juice

6 large eggs, separated, at room temperature

1/2 cup All Natural SomerSweet or sugar

2 teaspoons tangerine zest

1/4 cup heavy cream

Tangerine Crème Anglaise (recipe follows)

tangerine crème anglaise

PROTEIN, HEALTHY FATS

DETOX, LEVEL 1, LEVEL 2

6 large egg yolks

1³/4 teaspoons vanilla extract

1 teaspoon tangerine zest

2 cups heavy cream

1/2 cup All Natural SomerSweet or sugar

Whisk the egg yolks, vanilla, and tangerine zest in a bowl and set aside. Heat the cream in a saucepan over medium heat until hot but not boiling. Remove the cream from the heat and add the All Natural SomerSweet. Slowly pour the cream over the egg yolk mixture, whisking constantly. Return the mixture to the saucepan over low heat, whisking constantly until the mixture thickens and coats the back of a spoon. Serve warm or cover in an airtight container and refrigerate for 2 days. MAKES 2¹/2 CUPS

tiramisù

16 ounces mascarpone (or cream cheese), softened

¼ cup All Natural SomerSweet or sugar

1 teaspoon vanilla extract

1 cup strong brewed decaffeinated coffee

2 tablespoons unsweetened cocoa powder

2 cups heavy cream

18 Cocoa Meringue Cookies (page 347), not dipped into chocolate

2.5 ounces dark chocolate (at least 60% cocoa), grated

Beat together the mascarpone, All Natural SomerSweet, vanilla, and ¼ cup of the coffee with an electric mixer until smooth. Divide the mixture between two bowls. Add the cocoa powder to one bowl and beat until combined.

In a third bowl, beat the cream until stiff. Divide between the two bowls of mascarpone mixture. Fold in and set aside.

Place half of the cookies into an 8-inch square baking dish. Sprinkle with half of the remaining coffee. Spoon the chocolate cheese mixture over the cookies. Sprinkle with half the grated chocolate. Layer the rest of the cookies on top of the grated chocolate and sprinkle with the remaining coffee. Spread the last of the cheese mixture over the cookies. Sprinkle with the remaining grated chocolate. Cover and refrigerate 2 hours or overnight before serving. SERVES 6 TO 8

wild berry fool

1 cup heavy cream

¼ cup All Natural SomerSweet or sugar, or more to taste

1 pound mixed frozen berries, thawed and drained (strawberries, raspberries, blackberries, blueberries)

Fresh whole berries, for garnish

Place the cream and the All Natural SomerSweet in a mixing bowl and whip with an electric mixer until soft peaks form. Do not overbeat. Taste and add more SomerSweet if necessary.

Place the frozen berries in a food processor and pulse until the berries are chunky. Fold the berries into the whipped cream until well combined. Spoon into serving dishes and chill.

Garnish with the fresh berries before serving. SERVES 4

new york–style cheesecake

PROTEIN, HEALTHY FATS

DETOX, LEVEL 1, LEVEL 2

Preheat the oven to 350°F. Butter the sides and bottom of a 9-inch springform pan. Line the bottom with a double thickness of waxed paper. Lay two 24-inch-long pieces of aluminum foil on a work surface to make an X. Place the springform pan in the center of the foil and fold up around the sides to form a waterproof jacket.

In a large mixing bowl, beat the cream cheese and All Natural SomerSweet until light and fluffy. Add the eggs one at a time, beating well after each addition. Add the sour cream, lemon juice, lemon zest, and vanilla. Mix until smooth.

Pour the batter into the prepared pan and place in a large roasting pan. Place the roasting pan in the oven and pour enough hot water into the roasting pan to surround the cheesecake pan with 1 inch of water. (This is a water bath, which helps keep the cheesecake from cracking and curdling.)

Bake for 1 hour. Turn off the oven and let cool in the oven for an additional hour without opening the door. Remove the cheesecake from the water bath and cool to room temperature.

Cover and refrigerate the cheesecake in the springform pan, preferably overnight. To unmold, run a warm knife around the edges of the cheesecake before you release the springform. Transfer the cheesecake to a serving dish. SERVES 8 TO 10

Three 8-ounce packages cream cheese, at room temperature

$^3/_4$ cup All Natural SomerSweet or sugar

3 large eggs, at room temperature

1 cup sour cream

$1^1/_2$ tablespoons fresh lemon juice

1 teaspoon lemon zest

1 teaspoon vanilla extract

peppermint cheesecake with chocolate crust

PROTEIN, HEALTHY FATS, INSULIN TRIGGERS

LEVEL 1, LEVEL 2

CRUST

1½ cups unsweetened cocoa powder

½ teaspoon baking soda

¼ cup All Natural SomerSweet or sugar

8 tablespoons (1 stick) butter, chilled and cut into ½-inch pieces

1 large egg

1 teaspoon vanilla extract

FILLING

Three 8-ounce packages cream cheese, at room temperature

¾ cup All Natural SomerSweet or sugar

4 large eggs

1 cup heavy cream

2½ teaspoons pure peppermint extract

Chocolate Ganache (page 325), warmed

Preheat the oven to 275°F. Butter a 9-inch springform pan. Set aside.

For the crust: Place the cocoa powder, baking soda, All Natural SomerSweet, and butter into a food processor. Pulse until mixture resembles cornmeal. Add the egg and vanilla and pulse until mixture forms pea-size pieces. Pour into the prepared pan. Press into the bottom of the pan and set aside.

For the filling: In a large mixing bowl, beat the cream cheese and All Natural SomerSweet until light and fluffy. Add the eggs one at a time, beating well after each addition. Add the cream and peppermint extract. Mix until smooth.

Pour the filling into the prepared pan and place in a roasting pan or baking dish. Place the roasting pan in the oven and pour enough hot water into the roasting pan to surround the cheesecake pan with 1 inch of water. (This is a water bath, which helps prevent the cheesecake from curdling or cracking.) Bake for 1 hour. Without opening the oven door, turn off the heat and leave the cheesecake in the oven for an additional hour.

When the cheesecake is completely cooled, pour the warm chocolate topping over it, smoothing with a spatula. Cover and refrigerate overnight. Run a warm knife around the edges of the cheesecake before releasing the spring. Transfer the cheesecake to a serving dish.

SERVES 12

cappuccino cheesecake

PROTEIN, HEALTHY FATS

DETOX, LEVEL 1, LEVEL 2

Preheat the oven to 350°F. Butter the sides and bottom of a 9-inch springform pan. Line the bottom with a double thickness of waxed paper. Lay two 24-inch-long pieces of aluminum foil on a work surface to make an X. Place the pan in the center of the foil and fold up around the sides to form a waterproof jacket.

In a large mixing bowl, beat the cream cheese and All Natural SomerSweet until light and fluffy. Add the eggs one at a time, beating well after each addition. Add the sour cream and vanilla. Mix until smooth. Add the coffee and mix well.

Pour the batter into the prepared pan and place in a large roasting pan. Place the roasting pan in the preheated oven and pour enough hot water into the roasting pan to surround the cheesecake pan with 1 inch of water. (This is a water bath, which helps prevent the cheesecake from curdling or cracking.)

Bake for 1 hour. Turn off the oven and let the cheesecake cool in the oven for an additional hour without opening the door. Remove the cheesecake from the water bath and cool to room temperature.

Cover the cheesecake and refrigerate in the springform pan, preferably overnight. To unmold, run a warm knife around the edge of the cheesecake and transfer the cheesecake to a serving dish. Garnish with whipped cream and coffee beans. SERVES 8 TO 10

Three 8-ounce packages cream cheese, at room temperature

1 cup All Natural SomerSweet or sugar

3 large eggs, at room temperature

$^3/_4$ cup sour cream

1 tablespoon vanilla extract

$^1/_2$ cup strong brewed decaffeinated coffee

$^1/_2$ cup hot water

2 cups Perfectly Whipped Cream (page 317)

8 to 10 decaffeinated coffee beans

asian napoleons

Coconut oil, for frying

12 wonton skins

1 cup Vanilla Custard
(page 320)

8 to 10 large
strawberries, hulled
and thinly sliced

1 tablespoon ground
cinnamon mixed
with 2 tablespoons
All Natural
SomerSweet or
sugar

In a small saucepan, heat the oil to 375°F. If you don't have a thermometer to test your oil, use a small piece of wonton as a test. If the oil bubbles immediately when the wonton is added, it's hot enough.

Place a cookie sheet lined with paper towels on the counter next to the stove. Using tongs, place the wontons one at a time into the hot oil. Turn every few seconds, until the wonton starts to lightly brown. Wontons will continue to darken even when removed from oil. Be careful not to overcook. Remove each wonton from the oil and place on the paper towels. Then drain and blot excess oil.

Place 8 cooled wontons on a work surface. Spread or pipe about 1 tablespoon of custard on each wonton. Layer the strawberry slices on top of the custard. Dollop another tablespoon of custard on top of the strawberries.

Take 4 of the wontons layered with custard and berries and stack them on top of the 4 others. (Starting from the bottom, you should have wonton, custard, strawberries, custard, wonton, custard, strawberries, custard.) Then top each stack with the remaining 4 wontons to finish the napoleons.

Sprinkle each napoleon with the sweetened cinnamon and serve immediately.

MAKES 4 NAPOLEONS

chocolate-dipped cocoa meringue cookies

PROTEIN, CARBOHYDRATES, HEALTHY FATS

LEVEL 1, LEVEL 2

Preheat the oven to 250°F. Line a baking sheet with parchment paper and set aside.

Beat the egg whites and cream of tartar with an electric mixer until soft peaks form. Gradually add the All Natural SomerSweet while continuing to beat. Beat until the egg whites hold stiff peaks. Sift the cocoa powder onto the egg whites a little at a time. Fold in gently with a rubber scraper. Carefully fold in the grated dark chocolate.

Drop the batter by the spoonful or pipe the meringue from a pastry bag onto the prepared baking sheet. The cookies should be about 2 inches in diameter.

Bake the cookies for 1 hour. Turn the oven off. Leave the cookies in the oven with the door closed for an additional hour. Allow cookies to cool to room temperature. Peel cookies off parchment paper.

Dip the cookies halfway into the fudge sauce. Set on a cooling rack to dry before storing at room temperature in an airtight container. MAKES 18 COOKIES

5 egg whites, at room temperature

1/4 teaspoon cream of tartar

1 cup All Natural SomerSweet or sugar

3 tablespoons unsweetened cocoa powder

2.5 ounces dark chocolate (at least 60% cocoa), grated

1 recipe Dark Chocolate Fudge Sauce (page 316), warmed (omit for Level 1)

somersweet chocolate truffles

6 ounces unsweetened chocolate, chopped into small pieces

1½ cups heavy cream

¾ teaspoon vanilla extract

¾ cup All Natural SomerSweet or sugar

Pinch of baking soda

¼ cup unsweetened cocoa powder mixed with ¼ cup All Natural SomerSweet or sugar, for dusting finished truffles

Place the chopped chocolate in the bowl of a food processor or blender. Heat the cream in a saucepan over medium heat until small bubbles appear around the edge. Pour the cream over the chocolate and allow to stand for 30 seconds. Blend until the mixture is smooth. Add the vanilla, All Natural SomerSweet, and a pinch of baking soda. Transfer the mixture to a shallow dish and refrigerate until firm, at least 1 hour.

Using a 1-ounce scoop or a tablespoon, scoop balls of chocolate and place on a baking sheet. Refrigerate for about 30 minutes.

When chilled, roll each truffle in the palm of your hand into a perfect round ball. Drop the truffles into the sweetened cocoa powder to coat the exterior. Store the truffles in the refrigerator in an airtight container. MAKES ABOUT THIRTY 1-OUNCE TRUFFLES

ORANGE TRUFFLES Omit the vanilla and add ½ teaspoon orange extract.

CAPPUCCINO TRUFFLES Pour ¼ cup brewed decaf into the food processor or blender along with the chopped chocolate.

INDEX

RECIPE LIST

Watercress Mushroom Soup, 52 **gf ef**
Pumpkin Soup with Roasted Shallots and
Sage, 53 **gf df ef**
Split Pea Soup, 54 **gf ef v**
Tex-Mex Black Bean Soup, 55 **gf df ef v
vg**
Lentil Soup, 56 **gf df ef v vg**
Red Lentil Cumin Soup, 57 **gf df ef**
Cold Cucumber-Asparagus Soup, 58 **gf ef v**

SALADS

Arugula and Parmesan Salad, 61 **gf ef v**
Blue Cheese Vinaigrette with Crudités, 61
gf ef v
Garden Greens with Pear Tomatoes
and Lemon-Mint Vinaigrette, 62
gf df ef v vg
Iceberg Wedge with Roquefort Dressing,
62 **gf ef v**
Chopped Raw Zucchini and Parmesan
Salad, 63 **gf ef v**
Tricolore Salad with Balsamic Vinaigrette,
64 **gf df ef v vg**
Zucchini Carpaccio, 64 **gf ef v**
Baby Greens with Champagne Vinaigrette,
65 **gf df ef v vg**
Green Salad with Artichoke Hearts and Red
Wine Vinaigrette, 65 **gf df ef v vg**
Spinach Salad with Hot Bacon Dressing, 66
gf df
Buffalo Mozzarella, Fennel, and Celery
Salad, 67 **gf ef v**
Buffalo Mozzarella and Cherry Tomato
Salad, 67 **gf ef v**
Endive and Radicchio Salad with Stilton
Cheese, 68 **gf ef v**
Tomato and Cucumber Salad with Feta
Vinaigrette, 68 **gf ef v**
Maytag Blue Cheese and Roasted
Vegetable Salad, 69 **gf ef v**
Lamb's Lettuce Salad with Warmed Goat
Cheese, 70 **gf ef v**
Chanterelle Salad with Creamy Parmesan
Dressing, 71 **v**
Baby Spinach Salad with Vidalia Onions,
Sun-Dried Tomatoes, and Goat Cheese,
72 **gf ef**
Hearts of Palm and Artichoke Salad, 73
gf df ef v vg
Fennel, Red Onion, and Hearts of Palm
Salad, 73 **gf df v**
Israeli Salad, 74 **gf df ef v vg**

Green Bean Salad and Hearts of Palm, 74
gf ef v
Crunchy Cabbage Salad, 75 **gf df ef v vg**
Jícama and Snap Pea Citrus Salad, 75
gf df ef v vg
Crunchy Coleslaw, 76 **v**
Baby Greens with Sherry Shallot
Vinaigrette, 77 **gf df ef v vg**
Baby Artichoke Salad, 77 **gf ef v**
Asian Greens with Soy Vinaigrette, 78
df ef v vg
Greek Salad, 78 **gf ef v**
Broccoli and Cauliflower with Lemon-Garlic
Vinaigrette, 79 **gf df ef v vg**
Artichoke Bottoms with Dungeness Crab
Salad, 80 **gf df**
Apple Salad with Blue Cheese Vinaigrette,
80 **gf ef v**
Citrus-Marinated Barbecued Shrimp with
Fresh Arugula, 81 **gf df ef**
Spicy Rock Shrimp Salad, 82 **gf ef**
Salade Niçoise, 83 **gf df**
Warm Frisée Salad with Poached Egg and
Pancetta, 84 **gf df**
Cobb Salad, 85 **gf**
Caesar Salad, 86
Grilled Chicken Caesar Salad, 87
Parmesan Bowls with Caesar Salad, 87
Grilled Chicken Salad with Watercress and
Blue Cheese Vinaigrette, 88 **gf ef**
Grilled Chicken Salad with Sun-Dried
Tomatoes and Goat Cheese, 89 **gf ef**
Achiote Chicken with Radish and
Cucumber Salad, 90 **gf df ef**
Chopped Salami and Vegetable Salad, 91 **ef**
Taco Salad, 92 **gf ef**
Chopped Vegetable Salad with Roasted
Chicken, 93 **gf df ef**
Southern Country Fried Chicken Salad, 94
gf df
Chinese Chicken Salad, 95 **gf ef**
Pork Medallions over Pale Greens with
Pepper-Thyme Vinaigrette, 96 **gf df ef**
Warm Steak and Arugula Salad with
Parmesan Shavings, 97 **gf ef**
Thai Beef with Cucumber Salad, 98 **gf df
ef**
Tuna Salad in Lettuce Cups, 99 **gf df**
Turkey Salad in Lettuce Cups, 99 **gf df**
Tarragon Chicken Salad in Lettuce Cups,
100 **gf df**
Egg Salad in Lettuce Cups, 101 **gf df v**

Radicchio Cups with Curried Chicken, 102 **df**

Stay Sexy Forever!

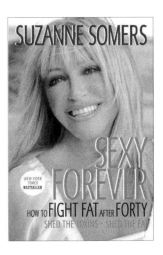

"Are you bloated? Sick of belly fat? Are your hormones out of whack?
It's not your fault! At a certain age, our bodies betray us. Diet and exercise alone just
don't cut it anymore. I've spent the past two decades working with a team of cutting-
edge doctors, and I've found the missing piece of the puzzle to losing weight after forty.
This new information will astonish you—and I want to share these discoveries with you
in my book *Sexy Forever!*" —Suzanne Somers

Whether you have just a few pounds to lose or are battling more,
this new plan will give you the knowledge you need to combat your toxic burden,
uncover hidden food allergies, and balance your hormones to become slim,
vibrant, healthy, and sexy . . . forever.

Sexy Forever
$15.00 paper (Canada: $17.00)
ISBN 978-0-307-58852-4

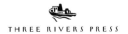

THREE RIVERS PRESS

AVAILABLE WHEREVER BOOKS ARE SOLD

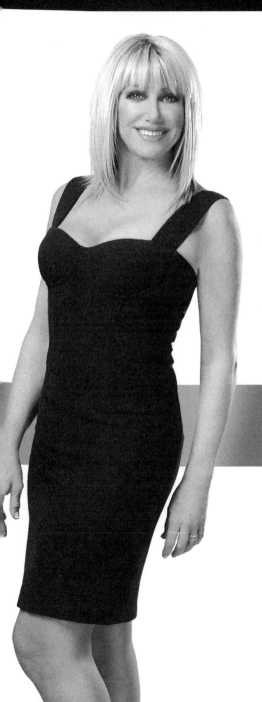